AF732904

CARDIOLOGY RESEARCH AND CLINICAL DEVELOPMENTS

ARTERIAL HYPERTENSION

ETIOLOGY, PATHOPHYSIOLOGY AND TREATMENT OPTIONS

Cardiology Research and Clinical Developments

Additional books in this series can be found on Nova's website under the Series tab.

Additional e-books in this series can be found on Nova's website under the e-book tab.

CARDIOLOGY RESEARCH AND CLINICAL DEVELOPMENTS

ARTERIAL HYPERTENSION

ETIOLOGY, PATHOPHYSIOLOGY AND TREATMENT OPTIONS

MARTEN VOSLER
AND
SIEMEN WEBER
EDITORS

New York

Copyright © 2013 by Nova Science Publishers, Inc.

All rights reserved. No part of this book may be reproduced, stored in a retrieval system or transmitted in any form or by any means: electronic, electrostatic, magnetic, tape, mechanical photocopying, recording or otherwise without the written permission of the Publisher.

For permission to use material from this book please contact us:
Telephone 631-231-7269; Fax 631-231-8175
Web Site: http://www.novapublishers.com

NOTICE TO THE READER

The Publisher has taken reasonable care in the preparation of this book, but makes no expressed or implied warranty of any kind and assumes no responsibility for any errors or omissions. No liability is assumed for incidental or consequential damages in connection with or arising out of information contained in this book. The Publisher shall not be liable for any special, consequential, or exemplary damages resulting, in whole or in part, from the readers' use of, or reliance upon, this material. Any parts of this book based on government reports are so indicated and copyright is claimed for those parts to the extent applicable to compilations of such works.

Independent verification should be sought for any data, advice or recommendations contained in this book. In addition, no responsibility is assumed by the publisher for any injury and/or damage to persons or property arising from any methods, products, instructions, ideas or otherwise contained in this publication.

This publication is designed to provide accurate and authoritative information with regard to the subject matter covered herein. It is sold with the clear understanding that the Publisher is not engaged in rendering legal or any other professional services. If legal or any other expert assistance is required, the services of a competent person should be sought. FROM A DECLARATION OF PARTICIPANTS JOINTLY ADOPTED BY A COMMITTEE OF THE AMERICAN BAR ASSOCIATION AND A COMMITTEE OF PUBLISHERS.

Additional color graphics may be available in the e-book version of this book.

Library of Congress Cataloging-in-Publication Data

ISBN: 978-1-62417-852-8

Library of Congress Control Number: 2012956340

Published by Nova Science Publishers, Inc. † New York

Contents

Preface

Arterial hypertension is one of the most frequent chronic diseases in the industrialized nations of the West and represents a major risk factor for cardiovascular morbidity and mortality. In this book, the authors present current research in the study of the etiology, pathophysiolgy and treatment options of arterial hypertension. Topics include endothelial dysfunction in hypertension; masked arterial hypertension; arterial hypertension in children and adolescence, treatment options, and influence of sex hormones; and target organ damage in hypertensive patients.

Chapter 1 – Introduction: The vascular endothelium plays an important rule in vascular homeostasis, tone and as a consequence, vascular health. Impairment in endothelial function or endothelial dysfunction translates to increased vascular tone and possibly to high blood pressure. Although is still debatable whether endothelial dysfunction remains a cause or consequence of essential hypertension, reversal of this target organ damage undoubtedly leads to improved cardiovascular prognosis. Not unreasonably, reversal of endothelial dysfunction has become therefore an ambitious treatment target. In this article, after exploring and providing evidence for the presence of endothelial dysfunction in hypertension, the authors also provide a systemic literature search review of endothelial dysfunction reversal in essential hypertension.

Methods: The authors conducted a MEDLINE, EMBASE etc. search of all of published studies referring to endothelial dysfunction reversal or improvement in hypertension from 1989 to 2012. Studies involving placebo were also included.

Results: The authors identified several pharmacologic and non-pharmacologic approaches favourably affecting endothelial function. Interestingly, blood pressure reduction per se did not affect vascular function. Modulators of the renin-angiotensin-aldosterone system (RAAS) appeared to have a consistent and a powerful effect in ameliorating or even reversing endothelial dysfunction in comparison to other antihypertensive agents for the same blood pressure control.

Conclusion: Reducing blood pressure without specific antihypertensive drugs does not seem to improve endothelial dysfunction. Modulators of the RAAS appear to have a long lasting beneficial effect on endothelial function perhaps providing a mechanistic link to their favourable effects on hypertensive cardiovascular prognosis.

Chapter 2 - In the early 2000s, masked hypertension (MAHT) was originally defined by Thomas Pickering as the hypertensive condition undetectable by conventional blood pressure

(BP) measurements in the clinic or office environment. Thus, MAHT is an elevated ambulatory or home BP in the absence of increased office BP.

The best way to diagnose MAHT is to use ambulatory BP monitoring (ABPM), because sleep-time BP can not be measured otherwise noninvasively. MAHT is an emerging clinical entity predisposing to subclinical organ damage and to increased cardiovascular risk.

MAHT prevalence has been estimated to be 10-38%. MAHT is prevalent and may be even more so: as home BP measurement becomes more popular, the detection MAHT will increase. MAHT is more frequently found in pre-hypertensive individuals. Recent study showed a MAHT prevalence of 8.1%; and older age, high-normal systolic and diastolic office BP, greater BMI, current smoking, diabetes, and electrocardiographic LVH were found to be independently correlated to MAHT.

According to some authors, there are basically two types of MAHT: 1) MAHT in general population (10-15%, which makes hundred millions in the world) in people with normal office BP, but elevated out-of-office BP (e.g. at workplace). 2) The other type of MAHT occurs in about 30% of patients with sustained ("classic") AHT, who have diagnosed AHT and apparently well-controlled BP (by therapy), i.e. normal office BP, but not normal BP all day long, e.g. BP is not controlled in the morning and/or in the night). Other authors believe that only the first type is MAHT, while the second is only "insufficiently efficient antihypertensive therapy."

Classification of MAHT into subtypes, according to BP circadian cycle (morning hypertension, daytime hypertension, and night-time hypertension regardless of the presence of antihypertensive treatment) has been recently proposed. MAHT carries nearly the same cardiovascular risks as sustained hypertension. In 2012 study, multivariate regression analyses revealed that the presence of MAHT was one of the independent determinants of LVH, carotid atherosclerosis, and albuminuria.

According to currently available medical literature, MAHT is prevalent, prognostically important, associated with subclinical damages and treatable form of hypertension, but insufficiently recognized entity.

Chapter 3 - Arterial hypertension is one of the most frequent chronic diseases in the industrialized nations of the West and represents a major risk factor for cardiovascular morbidity and mortality. The authors review the evidence on practice-based approaches to improving blood pressure control, from new styles of patient education to home blood pressure monitoring. The conventional antihypertensive therapies including renin–angiotensin–aldosterone system antagonists (converting enzyme inhibitors, receptor blockers, renin inhibitors, and mineralocorticoid receptor blockers), diuretics, β-blockers, and calcium channel blockers are variably successful in achieving the challenging target blood pressure values in hypertensive patients. Difficult to treat hypertension is still a commonly observed problem world-wide. A number of drugs are considered to be used as novel therapies for hypertension. Renalase supplementation, vasopeptidase inhibitors, endothelin antagonists, and especially aldosterone antagonists (aldosterone synthase inhibitors and novel selective mineralocorticoid receptor blockers) are considered an option in resistant hypertension. In addition, the aldosterone antagonists as well as (pro)renin receptor blockers or AT2 receptor agonists might attenuate end-organ damage. This array of medications has now been complemented by a number of new approaches of non-pharmacological strategies including vaccination, genomic interference, controlled breathing, baroreflex activation, and probably most successfully renal denervation techniques. It remains an exciting question which approach will confer the best blood pressure control and risk reduction in this tricky disease.

Chapter 4 - Sex hormones are steroids derived from cholesterol, which have numerous biological functions on reproductive organs, glands from these organs and on important systems of our organism controlling or modulating various functions such as reproduction, growth and metabolism. Moreover, the sex hormones are able to modulate blood pressure by acting on important systems as cardiovascular, renal and neural. These hormones can have either complementary or antagonistic actions. Indeed, it has been described in the technical literature that the actions of testosterone are contrary to the estrogen in the regulation of blood pressure. Estrogen alone or combined with progesterone has been associated with decreased blood pressure, whereas testosterone can raise blood pressure by stimulating the renin-angiotensin-aldosterone system. The effects of testosterone in the development of cardiovascular disease (CVD) are contradictory. While some researchers suggest positive effect, others indicate negative actions of testosterone. It has been reported that androgen deprivation in adult men impaired endothelium-dependent relaxation and promoted the progression of atherosclerosis. Nevertheless, many other clinical and epidemiological studies have also reported that testosterone inhibits CVD development. Another evidence about the benefits of the male sex hormone is laid down when the authors assessed the effects of induced hypogonadism on hypertension by analyzing large artery stiffening in men. Studies have shown that after three months of induced hypogonadism diastolic pressure is elevated, along with mean pulse pressure. Similarly, estrogen showed protective effects on vascular function and heart failure, which are related to the prevention of arterial hypertension. Estrogens can promote vasodilation and lower BP by different mechanisms as their direct actions on blood vessels, which physiologically stimulate the release of endothelium-derived vasodilator factors as well as modification of vasoconstrictor factors and inhibition of the renin-angiotensin system. Although the cardioprotective effects of estrogen are widely appreciated, little is known about the effects of progesterone, which is commonly used in hormone replacement therapy (HRT). Progesterone has both vasodilatory and vasoconstrictive effects in the vasculature depending on location of the vessel and level of exposure. Indeed, progesterone at physiological levels can inhibit the production of endothelin-1, but at supraphysiological levels, it inhibits endothelium-independent relaxation. Despite the alleged benefits of estrogen and progesterone on cardiovascular disease, the use of these hormones to postmenopausal women for HRT are still controversial. In addition, the negative findings of Heart and Estrogen/progestin Replacement Study (HERS) I and II and Women's Health Initiative (WHI) studies on HRT in postmenopausal women, such as stroke, venous thromboembolic disease and deep vein thrombosis have shaken the authors' previous ideas that HRT was protective. Thus, other therapies being tested in hormone replacement as the selective estrogen receptor modulator (SERMs) that, like estrogen, may induce endothelium-dependent acute vasodilation resulting in lowering of blood pressure. However, the mechanisms through which sex hormones modulate the blood pressure have not been fully elucidated. Therefore, the characterization of those could lead to a better understanding of hypertension in women and men, and perhaps to improved forms of therapy. In this chapter the authors will be a discussing the potential mechanisms through which male and female sex hormones may regulate the blood pressure as well as the cellular, biochemical and molecular pathways by which sex hormones may modify the effects of hypertension on the cardiovascular system.

Chapter 5 - This chapter will explore the importance of investigating the hypertension in childhood and adolescence that may emerge in adult life and debate a prevalence, incidence and occurrence of hypertension in children and adolescents, addition to addressing the methods and instruments used to determine hypertension, risk factors, health promotion, education and treatment for hypertensive children and adolescents.

Studies have shown significant rates of hypertension in children and adolescents and considering necessary to check blood pressure in childhood, since the increase in the arterial BP in youth indicates a prediction of hypertension in adulthood.

Studies involving analysis of hypertension risk factors should always register the prevalence and their correlations in childhood, as an essential to identify a population at risk. Therefore, the early detection of risk factors in asymptomatic children may contribute to a decrease in the development of hypertension and prevention of possible co morbidities.

In view of the substantial tracking of hypertension risk factors from adolescents to adulthood, there is an urgent need to intervene early with efficacious strategies to identify and treat hypertensive children and adolescents. The traditional hypertensive risk factors, namely overweight/obesity and family history, including lifestyle (a bad diet, stress, and insufficient physical activity) appear to be important, accounting for the dramatic recent changes in prevalence and would be of public health concern.

Chapter 6 - Hypertension should be considered a major risk factor for an array of cardiovascular and related diseases. Both systolic and diastolic blood pressures show a graded independent relationship with heart failure, peripheral artery disease and end stage renal disease. The 2003 ESH-ESC Guidelines emphasized that diagnosis and management of hypertension should be related to quantification of total (or global) cardiovascular risk. This concept is based on the fact that only a small fraction of the hypertensive population has an elevation of blood pressure alone, with the great majority exhibiting additional cardiovascular risk factors. Due to the importance of subclinical organ damage as an intermediate stage in the continuum of vascular disease and as a determinant of total cardiovascular risk, signs of organ involvement should be sought carefully by appropriate techniques:

- heart: electrocardiography and echocardiography should be part of all routine assessment of subjects with high BP;
- blood vessels: ultrasound scanning of carotid arteries is recommended when detection of vascular hypertrophy or asymptomatic atherosclerosis is deemed useful;
- kidney: diagnosis of hypertension-related renal damage is based on a reduced renal function or an elevated urinary excretion of albumin;
- fundoscopy: examination of eye grounds is only recommended in severe hypertensives;
- brain: silent brain infarcts, lacunar infarctions, microbleeds and white matter lesions are not infrequent in hypertensives, and can be detected by MRI or CT.

It is now clear that the stratification of cardiovascular risk through the assessment of organ damage is important for treating and reducing the risk of cardiovascular disease.

In: Arterial Hypertension
Editors: Marten Vosler and Siemen Weber
ISBN: 978-1-62417-852-8
© 2013 Nova Science Publishers, Inc.

Chapter 1

Endothelial Dysfunction in Hypertension: From Bench to Bedside and Future Directions

Ify Mordi[1], Natalie Sawdon[2] and Nikolaos Tzemos[1,*]
[1]Institute of Cardiovascular and Medical Sciences,
University of Glasgow, Glasgow, UK
[2]Renal Unit, Western Infirmary, Glasgow, UK

Abstract

Introduction: The vascular endothelium plays an important rule in vascular homeostasis, tone and as a consequence, vascular health. Impairment in endothelial function or endothelial dysfunction translates to increased vascular tone and possibly to high blood pressure. Although is still debatable whether endothelial dysfunction remains a cause or consequence of essential hypertension, reversal of this target organ damage undoubtedly leads to improved cardiovascular prognosis. Not unreasonably, reversal of endothelial dysfunction has become therefore an ambitious treatment target. In this article, after exploring and providing evidence for the presence of endothelial dysfunction in hypertension, we also provide a systemic literature search review of endothelial dysfunction reversal in essential hypertension.

Methods: We conducted a MEDLINE, EMBASE etc. search of all of published studies referring to endothelial dysfunction reversal or improvement in hypertension from 1989 to 2012. Studies involving placebo were also included.

Results: We identified several pharmacologic and non-pharmacologic approaches favourably affecting endothelial function. Interestingly, blood pressure reduction per se did not affect vascular function. Modulators of the renin-angiotensin-aldosterone system (RAAS) appeared to have a consistent and a powerful effect in ameliorating or even reversing endothelial dysfunction in comparison to other antihypertensive agents for the same blood pressure control.

* Address for Correspondence: Dr .Nikolaos Tzemos, Institute of Cardiovascular and Medical Sciences, University of Glasgow, BHF Glasgow Cardiovascular Research Centre, 126 University Avenue, Glasgow, G12 8TA; Telephone: +44 (0) 141 330 2079; Fax: +44 (0) 141 330 6997; E-mail: niko.tzemos@glasgow.ac.uk.

Conclusions: Reducing blood pressure without specific antihypertensive drugs does not seem to improve endothelial dysfunction. Modulators of the RAAS appear to have a long lasting beneficial effect on endothelial function perhaps providing a mechanistic link to their favourable effects on hypertensive cardiovascular prognosis.

1. The Vascular Endothelium: Anatomy and Physiology

The arterial wall consists of three layers: the adventitia (or tunica externa), the media and the intima, shown in Figure 1. The adventitial layer is made up of loosely tight connective tissue; specifically perivascular fibroblasts and collagen. In addition to the collagen it also contains a rich capillary blood supply and the autonomous nervous system terminals. The collagen gives the artery its stability and anchors it to nearby organs. The media is made up of smooth muscle cells (VSMC) and of a matrix of elastin, collagen and proteoglycans. It is well established that the arterial media layer has a double action: that of container and of damper. A function of container, because gives to the arterial wall its shape and also is responsible for keeping the blood within the vascular system, and a damping function, which is the phasic stress, produced by the elastic properties of the matrix and the tonic contracted or relaxed state of the smooth muscle cells. In addition to the vascular supportive measures, the VSMC also synthesises and matures collagen and the elastin of the extracellular matrix.

The intima is the innermost layer of the blood vessel. It is a single layer of endothelial cells lying on a support basement membrane called the internal elastic lamina. These vascular endothelial cells line every blood vessel in the body as well as the endocardium and are in direct contact with the luminal contents, i.e. blood. The endothelial cell surface in an adult human covers an extensive area and is composed approximately of 1 to 6 X 10^{13} cells and weights approximately 1 kg (Fishman 1982).

Since the pioneering work of Furchgott and Zawadzki [1], who identified that the large blood vessels of rabbits only relaxed in response to acetylcholine if the endothelium was intact, our concept of the endothelium and its functions over the last two decades has radically changed. Hence, rather than being thought of as an inert anatomical shelter, we now understand that the endothelium is actually a metabolically active endocrine, paracrine and autocrine organ with sustainable anti-atherogenic and anti-thrombotic properties. Indeed, one could say that taken altogether, it is the largest organ in the human body, even more so than the skin.

The vascular endothelium has numerous functions, which are summarised in table 1. Regarding hypertension, the most important role of the endothelium is it part in the regulation of vascular tone. The endothelium releases numerous substances with local (paracrine) action. These substances cause vasoconstriction or vasodilatation, and are summarised in table 2. The healthy endothelium is a natural inhibitor in its actions and is thus maintained in a natural state of predominant vasodilatation, and the most important substance for the maintenance of this state is nitric oxide (NO).

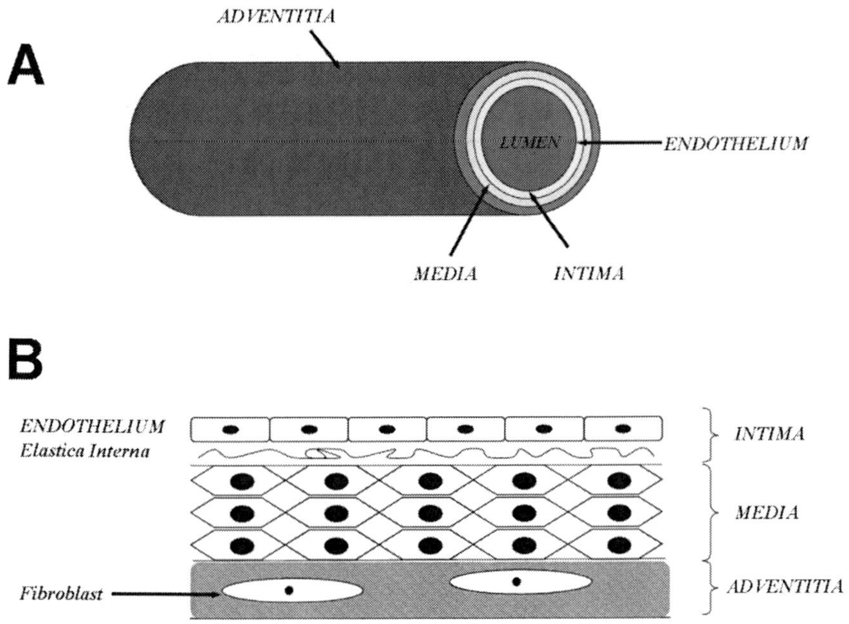

Figure 1. The structure of the human artery.

Table 1. Functions of the human vascular endothelium

Angiogenesis	Numerous growth factors affect the endothelium to cause the repair of old vessels and formation of new ones.
Barrier	The endothelium acts as a semi-selective barrier between the vessel lumen and surrounding tissue, controlling the passage of materials in and out of the bloodstream.
Clotting	The endothelium contains and secretes many pro-thrombotic and antithrombotic factors such as heparin sulphate (antithrombotic). It exists in naturally an antithrombotic state, which allows blood cells to roll along its surface.
Inflammatory	Mediation of inflammatory and immune responses.
Vascular tone	The endothelium contains substances that cause vasoconstriction and vasodilatation.

NO is a lipid and water soluble gas [2], formed by the conversion of the terminal guanidine-nitrogen from L-arginine, a semi-essential amino acid, to L-citrulline by an enzyme called endothelial NO synthase (eNOS), which is constitutive in endothelial cells (summarised in figure 2). There are three distinct isoforms of NO synthase: isoform I or nNOS (present in neuronal cells), isoform II or iNOS (in macrophages) which is calcium independent and cytokine-inducible and isoform III or eNOS originally described in the vascular endothelium but also present in platelets, myocardium and endocardium [3]. The activation of eNOS depends on the intracellular concentration of calcium ions in the endothelial cell, is calmodulin-dependent, and requires nicotinamide-adenine-dinucleotide (NADPH) and 5,6,7,8-tetrahydrobiopterin (BH4) as cofactors. Importantly, the activity of eNOS can be inhibited by endogenous and exogenous analogues of L-arginine such as NG-monomethyl-L-arginine (L-NMMA) and asymmetric dimethyl-arginine (ADMA), respectively [4, 5]. L-NMMA is an analogue of L-arginine that was initially shown to inhibit the generation of nitrite (NO2-) and nitrate (NO3-), which are products of the NO metabolism, in activated macrophages [6]. Subsequently, L-NMMA was also shown to induce contraction of vascular rings in isolated baths, an effect reversed by treatment with L- but not D-arginine [7].

Table 2. Some of the substances involved in maintenance of vascular tone

Endothelium Dependent Relaxing Factors	Endothelium Dependent Contracting Factors
Nitric oxide (NO)	Thromboxane A_2 (TxA_2)
Prostacyclin (PGI_2)	Endothelin
Endothelium derived hyperpolarising factor (EDHF)	Angiotensin II (AII)
C-type naturietic peptide (CNP)	

Once synthesised, part of the NO released diffuses directly to the underlying VSMC and relaxes them by stimulating a cytosolic enzyme, called soluble guanylate synthase. This activation leads to an increase in cyclic 3'-5'-guanisine monophosphate (cGMP) which is the second messenger, and to inhibition of the contractile apparatus, hence to vasodilatation. Apart from its conspicuous vasodilating properties, NO also inhibits VSMC proliferation and migration (hence preventing vascular remodelling) [8-10]. In addition, NO relaxes contractile elements in endothelial cells to preserve tight junctions and maintain impermeability [11]. However, the endothelial cells release NO not only abluminally to VSMC but also directly into the lumen. The part of NO released in the lumen interacts with circulating platelets and leukocytes inhibiting their adhesion [12]. Furthermore, NO acting synergistically with prostacyclin inhibits also platelet aggregation. However, nitric oxide has an extremely short half-life of only few seconds. Indeed, after synthesis, NO is rapidly inactivated by locally generated oxygen-derived free radicals (O_2^-) to form peroxynitrite anions ($OONO^-$) which have considerably less vasodilating capacity than NO. Because NO is a free radical itself, the chemical reaction between NO and superoxide anions is extremely fast, faster than that with superoxide dismutase (SODs) or with plasma vitamins which are natural scavengers of superoxide anions. Finally, part of NO released into the lumen is rapidly oxidised to nitrite and then to nitrate by oxygenated haemoglobin, molecular oxygen and superoxide anions and excreted as such in the urine [13].

NO synthesis and release is modulated by physical and humoral stimuli. The endothelial cells, because of their strategic anatomical position between the circulating blood and vascular smooth muscle, are exposed to continuous physical forces as shear stress, hydrostatic pressure and pulsatile stretch, particularly in the arterial circulation. Under resting conditions the interaction between endothelium and blood flow leads to mechanical endothelial changes and to subsequent NO release [14]. Moreover, it has been shown that changes in local flow also acutely increase NO release in vitro and contribute to flow-dependent vasodilatation in vivo [15]. The contribution of this basal NO release in peripheral vascular vasodilation was demonstrated by Vallance *et al* [5]. These authors have shown that in healthy subjects intra-arterial brachial administration of L-NMMA (a specific eNOS inhibitor) significantly reduced (up to a total of 40-45% from the basal forearm blood flow) the forearm blood flow in dose-dependent manner.

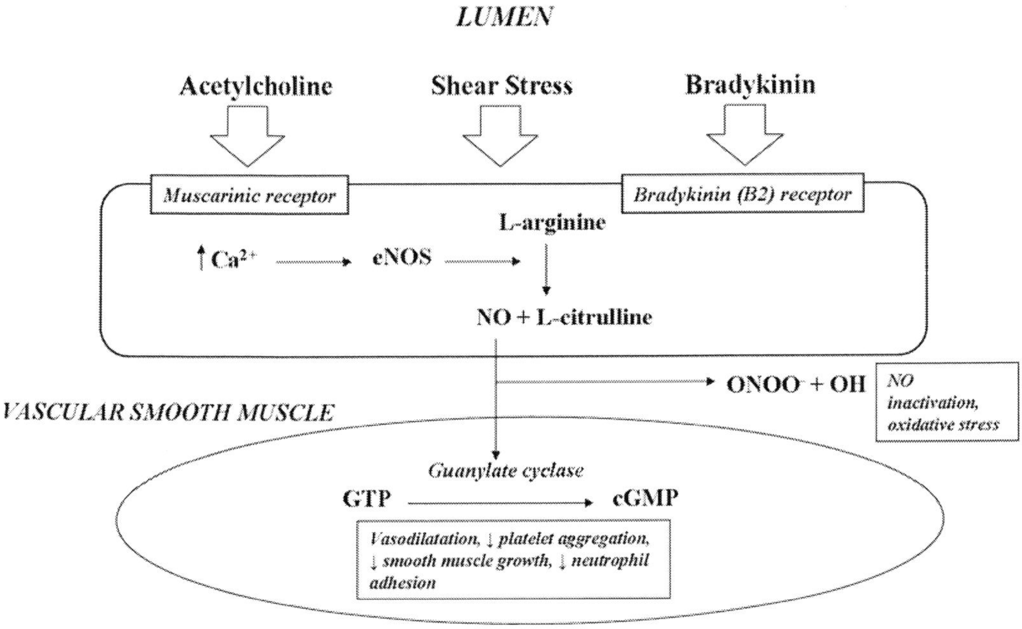

Figure 2. Synthesis of nitric oxide (NO).

Importantly, because L-NMMA is devoid of intrinsic constrictor activity on vascular smooth muscle cell and does not affect other systems on the arterial wall, its vasoconstrictive action on the arterial wall is endothelium-dependent suggesting that basal or tonic NO release plays a dominant role in the maintenance of peripheral vascular tone. Similarly, it has been shown that systemic L-NMMA infusion in animals and humans induced hypertensive responses predominantly by increasing vascular resistances [16, 17]. These hypertensive responses, although reversible by L-arginine, are not entirely attributed to increased vascular resistance. Indeed, an additional sodium-retaining mechanism might also contribute [18]. In contrast, basal release of NO does not appear to control the resting tone of peripheral veins, although it may have an effect in central veins [19].

Several neurohormonal mediators can cause 'stimulated' NO release through activation of specific endothelial receptors. Many substances have been identified as pharmacological NO agonists and few of them have constituted the pharmacological basis of investigating the L-arginine-NO pathway. Muscarinic agents such as acetylcholine, methylcholine and autacoids such as bradykinin and histamine remain the most frequently employed exogenous substances in assessing agonist-evoked endothelium-dependent vasodilation. Similarly, endogenous substances such as circulating hormones (catecholamines, vasopressin) and other mediators released by activated platelets [serotonin, adenosine diphosphate (ADP)] are able to stimulate NO release albeit by different coupling proteins. The endothelium releases other endothelium-dependent vasodilating factors (EDRF) such as prostacyclin [20] and the elusive endothelium-dependent hyperpolarizing factor (EDHF). In contrast, the endothelium also releases endothelium-derived contracting factors (EDCF) such as the peptide endothelin (ET-1), vasoconstrictor prostanoids (thromboxane A_2, prostaglandin H_2), superoxide anions and angiotensin II (Ang II). Finally, NO is known to be the mediator released in the peripheral nervous system by a complicated network of nerves, previously known as non-adrenergic and non-cholinergic [21, 22]. These nitrergic nerves are known to mediate vasodilation and regulation of blood supply to specific brain regions, by acting on the vascular smooth muscle cells[23]. However, their precise role and contribution in regulating blood pressure is not yet established [22].

Conceivably, the endothelium produces a host of substances clearly favouring those with endothelium-dependent vasodilating properties. The perennial release of NO from the endothelium also ensures additional antiatherogenic, antithrombotic and antiproliferative properties. In health, there is equilibrium between endothelial-derived vasodilating and endothelium-derived vasoconstricting substances favouring those with EDRF properties [24]. However, in several types of vascular disease, including hypertension, the endothelial cells become dysfunctional either structurally or functionally with a consequent impairment in evoking endothelium-dependent relaxations. This alteration is known as endothelial dysfunction and is mainly caused by either a reduction in release and/or increased inactivation and hence bioactivity of EDRF, although an additional excessive and unopposed release of EDCF's may also contribute.

2. Endothelial Dysfunction in Hypertension

The theory for development of hypertension from endothelial dysfunction is clear: we have already seen that dysfunctional endothelium is unable to dilate. We also know that there is a four-fold relationship between lumen diameter and flow. Taking this into consideration, it would be easy to assume that a dysfunctional endothelium would lead to an increase in blood pressure. However, the evidence for this is not entirely definitive; indeed, there is evidence to suggest that hypertension itself may cause hypertension.

Hypertension is a process characterised by elevated arterial blood pressure and its long-term sequelae on target organs leads to a considerably high cardiovascular mortality and morbidity [25]. The changes occurring during the hypertensive process on the wall of the resistant arteries are crucial determining and also perpetuating the hypertensive process itself. Indeed, in response to the increased arterial pressure the vessel structure is actively modified via a process known as vascular remodelling. This vascular process includes an active rearrangement of cellular and non-cellular elements involving elements both in intima and media layers (remodelling) around a smaller lumen [26]. In contrast, the process known as vascular hypertrophy, which involves VSMC proliferation, hypertrophy, and/or poliploidy, is thought to occur throughout the vessel [26, 27]. Therefore, this pressure-induced active restructuring of the arterial wall induces marked changes in luminal vascular dimensions, which along with alteration in endothelial cell shape and dimension results in elevated peripheral vascular resistance. Elevated peripheral vascular resistance, which is the hallmark of hypertension, is not an isolated phenomenon to be found only in macrocirculation but also in microcirculation [28]. Although, the mechanism by which this active remodelling is achieved is not completely understood, the endothelium might have a leading role.

Because of its strategic position within the vascular wall, the endothelium acts both as a 'sensor' detecting signals due to changes in haemo- and humoral factors, and also as a 'transducer' and 'mediator' of these signals. For example, in a condition where an increased flow is achieved (e.g. arterio-venous fistula), the luminal diameter of the artery is increased [29]. In contrast, in conditions with reduced blood flow the lumen diameter is decreased [30]. It is now well established that these vascular homeostatic functions are mediated by the endothelium and in particular via shear stress [31]. However, in hypertension shear stress is only minimally affected whilst in contrast circumferential stretch and/or tension are greatly increased [32]. This increased vascular wall tension promotes the release of vasoconstrictive agents such as EDCFs and PDGF as well as matrix modulators such as collagen [33, 34]. Hence, increased vascular wall stretch and tension will potentially promote vascular hypertrophy and/or formation of myoproliferative lesions, creating a vicious circle. Furthermore, endothelial cells regulate vascular tone, haemostasis, inflammation, cell growth, cell migration and interactions with the extracellular matrix through many receptor-mediated mechanisms. It is now well established that vascular growth factors interacting with specific receptors mediate part of the vascular remodelling in hypertension. In particular, structural changes such as VSMC hypertrophy are mediated partly by an increase of growth factors such as TGF-β1, but also by increased local activation of neurohormones as angiotensin II [35, 36]. In addition, increased matrix proteinases as collegenase and elastase are responsible for the lamellae fragmentation and their consequent replacement by collagen and elastin [37]. Similarly, it has been hypothesised that an increase of VSMC might also amplify the vasoconstrictive response to neurohormones thus further increasing systemic vascular resistance, hence blood pressure [38]. A part from structural changes, it is now accepted that an equal (if not superior) contribution to develop and maintain high peripheral vascular resistances in hypertension is given by functional arterial wall changes.

An impairment of NO bioactivity was initially confirmed in animal models of hypertension in the late 80's. These initial experiments were based on the observation of impaired vascular responses to pharmacological agonists of NO dependent vasodilatation in hypertensive animals [20, 39, 40]. Of particular interest in those initial animal studies was the fact that the degree of impairment of agonist-induced NO release was positively correlated to the level of arterial BP and antihypertensive treatment was able to improve these impaired vascular responses [41-44]. Furthermore, in spontaneous hypertensive rats (SHR) it was shown that the impairment in agonist (ACh) induced vasodilation was secondary to an imbalance between endothelium-dependent vasodilation and vasoconstrictors favouring the latter [45, 46].

In humans, the first demonstration of impaired endothelial dysfunction in hypertensive patients was first reported in the forearm resistance vessels in the early 90's by Panza et al [47]. Since this first report a plethora of studies by independent researchers also confirmed the presence of endothelial dysfunction in primary and secondary hypertension and also in various vascular territories. Furthermore, it was also confirmed that the abnormality in endothelial-dependent vasodilation was not confined only to the muscarinic receptor level, since acetylcholine was principally deployed as pharmacological NO-agonist, but also extended to other NO evoked agonists [48]. Similarly, the basal NO release assessed by L-NMMA infusion was found also to be blunted in hypertensive patients [49, 50] compared to normotensive controls. In contrast, the endothelium-independent vasoconstricting and vasodilating vascular responses were found to be similar in hypertensive and control groups arguing against an intrinsic alteration of VSMC responsiveness in hypertension [50, 51]. Although, there is overwhelming evidence to suggest the presence of endothelial dysfunction in hypertension, this is not a universal finding. To date only two studies have argued the presence of endothelial dysfunction in hypertension [52, 53]. The discrepancies between those two studies and the rest cannot be clearly explained, suggesting a complex and intriguing mechanism of endothelial dysfunction in hypertension.

The dysfunction of the endothelium is not limited to a reduction in production in NO however. A process called oxidative stress also leads to increased consumption of NO and contributes to an increase in vascular tone. Normal healthy endothelial cells produce dangerous reactive oxygen species (free radicals). The production of these free radicals is normally balanced by their elimination; however, in endothelial dysfunction the production far outweighs their removal [54-56]. Nitric oxide (an anion), after synthesis, is rapidly inactivated by locally (of endothelial and extra-endothelial origin) generated oxygen-derived free radicals ($O^{-}2$) to form peroxynitrite anions ($OONO^{-}$), which have considerably less vasodilating capacity than NO [57, 58]. The chemical reaction between NO and superoxide anions is extremely fast, faster than that with superoxide dismutase (SODs) or with plasma vitamins which are natural scavengers of superoxide anions. An increase in free-radical formation otherwise known as oxidative stress is present in many cardiovascular diseases including hypertension, hyperlipidaemia and heart failure [59-62]. Interestingly, the severity of hypertension appears to correlate with the degree of underlying oxidative stress [63]. Antioxidants, whether endogenous or exogenous in origin are part of an additional scavenging mechanism directed to "overcome" the excess of superoxide anion production. Hypertension has been described as a disease characterised by an excess of oxygen free radicals coupled with an inefficient antioxidant mechanism [61, 64, 65]. There is evidence to suggest that hypertensive patients have significantly lower plasma concentrations of naturally occurring antioxidant factors (thiols, vitamins A, C, E) compared with matched normotensive volunteers [61, 65]. Also, free radical scavengers such as superoxide dismutase (SOD), and glutathione (GSH) are reported to be depressed in hypertensive patients [66, 67]. It appears however, that overall NO is of vital importance to the endothelial dysfunction in hypertension.

3. Clinical Implications of Endothelial Dysfunction in Hypertension

Since there is ample evidence to suggest that NO regulates vascular tone, researchers have focused their interest on the appealing hypothesis of endothelial dysfunction being the promoter of the hypertensive process. Similarly, because NO has vasodilatory and additional anti-atherogenic properties, decreased bioavailability of NO may contribute to the increased peripheral vascular resistance and also provide a link between hypertension and its most important complication, the development of atherosclerosis. This hypothesis was further reinforced by the discovery that systemic administration of the L-arginine analogue L-NMMA induced sustained hypertension both in human and animal models [17], primarily by modulating vascular resistance. Although, it is yet unclear whether endothelial dysfunction is a cause or a consequence of hypertension, there are some intriguing associations between impaired NO bioactivity and hypertension.

The findings of the Framingham study have suggested that hypertensive patients had a twice fold increased risk of cardiovascular death to that of the non-hypertensive population. Since endothelial dysfunction is present before any structural irregularities in the arterial wall [68] it is conceivable that this represents the first vascular target organ damage en route to developing atherosclerosis. Furthermore, the confirmation that endothelial dysfunction was ubiquitous in diverse vascular territories in patients with hypertension led to intriguing speculation on the strong association between hypertension and cardiovascular morbidity and mortality. Brush *et al* [69] first showed that hypertensive patients with angina pectoris had a significant reduction in maximal coronary vasodilation (coronary reserve) to pharmacological agents and also myocardial ischaemia without any evidence of atherosclerosis or left ventricular hypertrophy. Therefore, in those patients the 'classical' aetiology of ischaemia by obstructive and/or extrinsic vascular compression of the epicardial arteries by the hypertrophied myocardium was debated. Similarly, Treasure *et al* [70] later observed that whilst in normal (morphologically smooth) epicardial coronary arteries the muscarinic agonist acetylcholine (ACh) caused NO release and thus vasodilatation; in subjects with hypertension the same agent caused paradoxical vasoconstriction. Brush *et al* [69] also observed a similar 'paradoxical' vasoconstrictive intracoronary response to ACh in hypertensive patients without left ventricular hypertrophy. Importantly, the vascular vasodilatory response to nitroglycerine (a NO donor) in both studies was not different between normotensive and hypertensive group of patients. Treasure *et al* showed that the presence of left ventricular hypertrophy in hypertensive patients was strongly associated with coronary endothelial dysfunction and Egashira *et al* [71, 72] showed that this abnormal (vasoconstrictive) epicardial response was not limited to the muscarinic agonists but also included substance P. Hence, we can speculate that the presence of impaired endothelial dysfunction at the coronary level in hypertensive patients, even in those without any significant obstructive disease, critically limits the coronary reserve therefore creating a potential source for ischaemia, especially in situations where high metabolic demand is required. Furthermore, the presence of endothelial dysfunction at the coronary level might also explain the discrepancy between angiographically normal coronary arteries and occurrence of cardiac chest pain [73] and/or acute coronary syndromes seen in hypertensive and normotensive patients with cardiovascular risk factors [74].

Ghiadoni *et al* [75] have shown that the presence and degree of agonist-evoked endothelium-dependent vasodilation in hypertensives was highly (inversely) correlated to common carotid artery intima-to-media wall ratio. Intima to media wall ratio is a good surrogate marker of atherosclerosis [76] and also correlates (though weakly) to concomitant coronary atherosclerosis [77].

Left ventricular hypertrophy (LVH) is a cardinal manifestation of preclinical cardiovascular disease [78] that strongly predicts future myocardial infarction, stroke, and cardiovascular death in patients with hypertension [79] and also in members of the general population [25, 80]. It has been shown that the risk of death or non-fatal implications, particularly ischaemic vascular events, is increased by to two- to fourfold in the presence of LV hypertrophy, independently of age, gender and other risk factors. Interestingly, although the prognostic significance of hypertensive left ventricular hypertrophy is well established, the mechanism of the adverse association between high LV mass and vascular events has not been well established. The evidence that LVH is associated with an increased systemic arterial wall thickness [81, 82] and more pronounced systemic atherosclerosis [83] has led to the speculation that those changes are also affecting the coronary microcirculation hence limiting coronary reserve. Perticone *et al* [84] showed that acetylcholine-evoked endothelium-dependent vasodilation in the forearm microcirculation of never-treated hypertensive patients with echocardiographic left ventricular hypertrophy was inversely related to LV mass and was significantly blunted as compared to normotensive volunteers. Similar results were also obtained by Millgard *et al* [85] suggesting a probably significant contribution of endothelial dysfunction in determining LVH, which leads to increased cardiovascular risk.

There is evidence suggesting a significant correlation between the degree of endothelial dysfunction and the severity of high blood pressure in hypertensive patients. Von zur Muhlen *et al* [86] investigated the relationship between ambulatory blood pressure and endothelium-dependent vasodilation in 25 untreated hypertensives. They showed that both 24-hr ambulatory blood pressure and office BP related inversely to the degree of endothelial-dependent vasodilation whilst there was no correlation with endothelium-independent vascular responses. Forte *et al* [87] found a strong inverse correlation between mean arterial blood pressure and urinary nitrite and nitrate (index of NO synthesis) in hypertensive patients. Conversely, two independent studies conducted in the normal population found that age, cholesterol, BMI but not BP were significantly related to endothelium-dependent vasodilation [88, 89].

Evidence has now begun to appear confirming the adverse prognostic value of endothelial dysfunction. In several recent studies, the presence of endothelial dysfunction strongly predicted future cardiac outcome [90-92]. The study by Halcox et al looked at coronary endothelial dysfunction in 308 patients and found that endothelial dysfunction was in fact more predictive of future coronary adverse events than the apparent angiographic severity of any lesion seen. Further studies have also demonstrated the prognostic significance of brachial artery endothelial dysfunction in predicting cardiovascular mortality [93, 94]. These results were mirrored by Yeboah et al [95] examined FMD in 2792 older patients (age 72-98 years). The authors found that event-free survival was significantly higher in patients with an FMD higher than the median compared to those lower than the median. Again, endothelial dysfunction was an independent predictor of future cardiovascular events. Interestingly, there have also be a couple of studies looking at endothelial dysfunction in patients with risk factors for coronary disease but no prior diagnosis. A study conducted by Perticone et al [96] examined 225 patients with untreated hypertension looking at brachial artery endothelial function and followed up for cardiovascular events. Endothelial function was measured by looking at arterial response (by forearm blood flow) to acetylcholine infusion. The authors found that the only independent predictors of future cardiovascular events were mean 24-hour blood pressure and endothelial dysfunction as measured by forearm blood flow response. Modena et al [97] examined 400 women with hypertension and impaired FMD and gave them 6 months of anti-hypertensive therapy. In the group in which there was no change in endothelial dysfunction there were over twice as many adverse cardiovascular events compared to those in who FMD improved, a statistically significant difference. Finally, Anderson et al [98] in the long-term follow up of the FATE study found that hyperemic velocity was a significant predictor of future cardiovascular events. Hyperemic velocity is a novel measure of blood flow velocity at hyperemia during an FMD examination and has been suggested to be more predictive or future cardiovascular adverse events than FMD alone [99].

It is conceivable that endothelial dysfunction represents a common pathway to all cardiovascular disease whereby, independently of the cause, this leads to atherosclerosis – this hypothesis is being increasingly backed up by the evidence.

4. Reversal of Endothelial Function in Human Hypertension

4.1. Strategies for Improving Endothelial Dysfunction in Hypertension

As we have discussed earlier in the chapter, a functionally and structurally intact endothelium has anti-atherogenic, anti-atherosclerotic and anti-proliferative properties. Thus, in theory an improvement of endothelial dysfunction would further improve cardiac prognosis in hypertensive patients making it an attractive therapeutic target. Hypertension is of course not just about reducing the raw blood pressure figures, but its management should include multiple risk factors intervention, and endothelial dysfunction should also probably be considered as a modifiable risk factor. There is clear evidence suggesting that reducing blood pressure in hypertension is much less effective in lowering coronary events than in lowering cerebral events [100]. This might be because drug treatment that reduces blood pressure might have no impact on the underlying endothelial dysfunction. In other words, although most hypertensives have endothelial dysfunction, most therapies that reduce blood pressure may not improve endothelial dysfunction meaning that, endothelial dysfunction may persist despite adequate control of clinic blood pressure. Because endothelial dysfunction precedes atherosclerosis, ensuring its reversal may well reduce the "coronary shortfall" and hence be a crucial missing link between hypertension and cardiovascular mortality. In this chapter we explore whether this could be true. Firstly, we will discuss non-pharmacological methods to improve endothelial dysfunction.

4.2. Exercise

Exercise is recognised as an effective non-pharmacological measure that reduces BP [101-103]. Regular (at least 3 times/week) aerobic exercise of moderate intensity reduces blood pressure by an average of 4/3mmHg. Exercise is recommended as an integral part of the international guidelines in primary and secondary prevention of hypertension [104]. Kokkinos *et al* [102] have previously shown that moderately intense aerobic exercise reduced significantly both systolic (average 7mmHg) and diastolic BP (average 5mmHg) in Afro-Caribbean patients with severe hypertension. In the same study, regression in left ventricular hypertrophy was also achieved. Since basal NO release is facilitated by constant shear stress, it has been postulated that regular exercise increases laminar flow and increases shear stress and hence NO release [105]. The beneficial effects of exercise on endothelial function in hypertensive patients have been confirmed by Higashi *et al* [106]. This group showed that 12 weeks of aerobic exercise, such as walking for 30min, 5 to 7 times per week, improved stimulated (acetylcholine-induced) NO release in previously untreated hypertensives. Interestingly, along with a significant reduction in blood pressure (7/4mmHg), there was also an associated significant reduction in LDL with an increase in HDL. A reduction in circulating LDL might act as a co-factor in improving both endothelial function and reducing BP. Total and LDL cholesterol have been correlated inversely with NO bioactivity both in healthy and in hypertensive subjects [88, 107]. This relationship is probably related to oxidized LDL and its ability to interfere with both NO formation and its inactivation [108, 109].

The results of Hambrecht *et al* [110] on the effect of exercise on the coronary vasculature are of particular note. This group showed that regular and programmed exercise improved stimulated NO release (acetylcholine-induced) in patients with established coronary artery disease. This suggests that a simple and moderate exercise program could potentially modify the coronary artery disease process. Indeed, this hypothesis has been recently tested and proven to be correct by Cornelissen et al [111] who studied endothelial function in 146 patients with stable coronary artery disease who were enrolled in a cardiac rehabilitation program. After twelve weeks there was a mean increase in FMD of 37% (although interestingly there was no improvement in reactive hyperemia index as measured by applanation tonometry). Beyond the effective of exercise on NO, several studies have also suggested an anti-inflammatory effect, reducing the numbers of circulating pro-inflammatory cytokines and CRP. CRP has been shown to have some atherosclerotic properties [112] and elevated levels are a predictor for adverse cardiovascular events [113]. Milani et al [114] found that an extended cardiopulmonary exercise programme ("cardiac rehabilitation") caused a significant drop in high-sensitivity CRP (42% compared to control). A further study by Vona et al [115] found that 4 weeks aerobic training provided improvement in endothelial function, either on its own or combined with resistance training. Interestingly, after 1 month of detraining the effect was lost, suggesting that exercise must be continued to have persistent benefit.

There is increasing evidence to suggest that exercise improves markers of endothelial dysfunction. The methods by which it does this are not yet fully understood however, and this remains an interesting area for further research.

4.3. Other Cardiovascular Risk Factors Associated with Hypertension

Endothelial dysfunction in hypertension is worsened by coincidental risk factors with known pro-atherogenic potential such age, total and LDL cholesterol, cigarette smoking, and gender [71, 88, 107, 116]. Taddei et al [107, 117] found that ageing was associated with progressively impaired NO bioactivity, and in hypertensives, endothelial dysfunction was accelerated with ageing. This group also reported a bimodal relationship between ageing and endothelial dysfunction. In the younger age group (18-30 years) the mechanism of endothelial dysfunction appeared to be related to a relative deficiency of L-arginine (substrate of NO) whereas in later life (>45 years) a cyclooxygenase-dependent mechanism was more apparent. Al-Shaer et al [118] obtained similar results comparing patients over 60 with atherosclerosis to those over 60 without and young healthy controls using venous occlusion plethysmography. The authors found that there was a significantly higher response in forearm blood flow in the younger group compared to both elderly groups. The group of elderly patients without atherosclerosis were free of all other cardiovascular risk factors, suggesting that age in itself plays a part in endothelial dysfunction. While the process behind which ageing causes endothelial dysfunction is not entirely understood, there is an increasing belief that it is caused by a combination of oxidative stress, reactive oxygen species and an increase in inflammatory cytokines [119]. Furthermore, the endothelium is naturally always in a state of repair and regeneration. As we age, mutations accumulate during the process of mitosis, leading to a slowing of this process. Eventually, the cells become senescent i.e. unable to divide and repair themselves anymore, again contributing to endothelial dysfunction [120]. This of course can be exacerbated by other factors.

Hyperlipidaemia is associated with increased oxidative stress, which adversely affects endothelial NO release [121, 122]. Apart from chronically elevated cholesterol, even a single high-fat meal also transiently impairs stimulated NO release, an effect that can last for up to 6 hours post-prandially [123]. More importantly it has recently been shown that even subjects with normal to high cholesterol levels have endothelial dysfunction [124]. Muiesan et al [125] looked at the effects of "generic" blood pressure lowering treatment in patients with hypertension and a total cholesterol of >6 mmol/L (mean 6.33). They found that with adequate BP control, irrespective of type of drugs used, forearm reactive hyperaemia was improved after 12 months of treatment. More specifically, Okumura et al [126] have recently found that small low-density lipoprotein (LDL) cholesterol was an independent predictor of endothelial dysfunction in 120 men. Conversely, low levels of high-density lipoprotein (HDL) cholesterol have been shown to be predictive of adverse cardiovascular risk [127] even if LDL levels are low [128]. Administration of reconstituted HDL cholesterol has been shown to improve endothelial function in several studies [129-131]. This effect has also been reproduced in diabetic patients with natural HDL ([132]). Furthermore, Sorrentino et al also gave the patients in their study niacin, which incrementally increased the beneficial effects of HDL cholesterol.

Cigarette smoking, whether active or passive causes oxidative stress which is associated with impaired NO release [133-135]. Additionally, smoking also causes a pro-inflammatory state with an increase in leukocytes and inflammatory cytokines, adding to endothelial dysfunction [136, 137]. Gender and race also have important impact on functional integrity of the endothelium [138, 139]. There is the general tendency to exclude pre-menopausal women from vascular endothelial function studies because of the confounding effects of oestrogens on the endothelium pre-menopause [140-142]. Virdis et al [143] compared the vascular effects of acetylcholine, L-NMMA and vitamin C in healthy women with leiomyoma pre- and post oophorectomy. They found that acute endogenous oestrogen deprivation (oophorectomy) was associated with endothelial dysfunction via a reduction in NO availability and this was restored by oestrogen replacement therapy.

The above-described factors are all capable of initiating and promoting endothelial dysfunction on their own, but their combined vascular effects with high blood pressure have not being investigated. In current management guidelines, patients with coronary artery disease are being treated with a more holistic approach, which address all the concomitant risk factors. This will hopefully lead to improved coronary artery endothelial function. As discussed earlier, there are now long-term data to suggest that endothelial dysfunction of the coronary arteries can predict outcome [90].

4.4. Anti-hypertensive Treatment

Whether endothelial dysfunction is a cause or a consequence of hypertension has long been debated. The evidence that impaired NO bioactivity pre-exists in the normotensive offspring of hypertensive patients, 20-30% of who will later develop hypertension, points towards the probable primary nature of this phenomenon [144-146]. If, however, endothelial dysfunction were the consequence of the hypertensive process then one would expect normalisation of BP should reverse this abnormality, however, this is clearly not the case. Panza et al [147] showed that adequate BP control with antihypertensive treatment (mainly with beta-blockers/diuretics) did not affect NO bioactivity in the forearm resistance circulation of patients with hypertension. The failure of "first-line" drugs to improve endothelial function supports the notion that endothelial dysfunction is the cause rather than the consequence of hypertension. Alternatively, Millgård and Lind [148] showed that blood pressure rise in itself can impair the endothelial function in that noradrenaline infusion caused both blood pressure rise and impaired stimulated NO release in forearm vasculature of healthy normotensive volunteers. Although the impairment in NO release observed in their study could have been the consequence of complex interaction between norepinephrine and the endothelium rather a pure rise in BP, Paniagua et al [149] have recently addressed this issue. They obtained similar results on stimulated NO release of small resistance vessels (subcutaneous) in normotensive humans after transient elevation of intravascular hydrostatic pressure. Furthermore, at least in secondary hypertension, removal of the underlying cause (aldosterone-producing adenomas) reverses endothelial dysfunction and also normalises blood pressure [150]. Hence the interaction between endothelial dysfunction and blood pressure might be more complex than simply saying that one must cause the other. In support of this hypothesis, Panza speculated that there are some hypertensive patients where endothelial dysfunction precedes high blood pressure. It could well be that endothelial dysfunction is both a cause and a consequence of hypertension i.e. a vicious circle might exist between endothelial dysfunction and elevated blood pressure.

4.4.1. Beta-blockers and Diuretics

Beta-blockers and thiazide diuretics are commonly prescribed therapies for hypertension. Despite their proven efficacy in improving overall prognosis in hypertension, they appear not to affect the NO-L-arginine pathway [125, 151-153]. One exception is nebivolol, a highly selective $\beta 1$-blocker that has been shown to improve endothelial dysfunction both in vivo and vitro [154, 155]. Dawes et al [156] reported that acute intra-arterial administration of nebivolol improved forearm vasculature NO bioactivity in hypertensive patients. Although the mechanism by which nebivolol improves endothelial dysfunction in hypertension is not yet fully elucidated a putative pharmacological cross-reactivity between serotonin and β-receptors might potentially explain these vascular effects [157]. Kakoki et al [158] showed that 5-HT1 blockade with a specific antagonist almost abolished the vasodilatory response to nebivolol in the rat kidney preparation, suggesting some receptor mediated interaction. Also, a possible antioxidant property of nebivolol has been suggested as an additional factor increasing NO-bioactivity or even a reduction in endothelin (ET-1) release [159, 160]. The beneficial effects of nebivolol on the endothelium were confirmed in humans by Tzemos et al [161]. In a double-blind crossover trial, 12 hypertensive patients were given 8 weeks of treatment with bendroflumethiazide plus atenolol or nebivolol (and then switched to the other group). With both treatments the blood pressure reduction was the same, however there was a significant increase in both forearm vasodilatory response to acetylcholine and the vasoconstrictor response to L-NMMA, suggesting that there may be a beneficial effect of nebivolol beyond a simple blood pressure reduction. The endothelial effects of nebivolol are unique amongst beta-blockers. For example, carvedilol, which is recommended in heart failure, does not mediate its beneficial effects in that condition by any improvement in endothelial function [162]. Indeed, the tide has recently turned against beta-blockers as first line treatment for hypertension due to poorer outcomes compared with other blood-pressure lowering medications [163-165]. Given the similar anti-hypertensive effects of nebivolol compared with atenolol however [161, 166], it is certainly of interest to investigate outcomes with nebivolol to see if there is an incremental benefit over and above other beta-blockers.

Recently, Sorrentino et al [167] conducted a study in mice with iatrogenic extensive anterior myocardial infarctions and were randomised to nebivolol, metoprolol or placebo. Although infarct size and heart rate was the same in both groups, left ventricular ejection fraction was significantly higher at 4 weeks in the nebivolol group (32% vs. 17% vs. 19%; $p < 0.05$) and survival was higher in the nebivolol group compared to the placebo group. Furthermore, there was a decrease in left ventricular adverse remodelling in the nebivolol group compared to metoprolol as judged by a more pronounced inhibition of myocyte hypertrophy. The authors felt that this may have been mediated by inhibition of cardiac NADPH oxidase by nebivolol (but not metoprolol), which had also been seen in mouse studies by Doerries and Looi [168, 169]. Nebivolol seems to have beneficial effects on smooth muscle cell proliferation, gene expression and oxidative stress [170, 171].

It seems that there is increasing evidence to support the theory that nebivolol has additional beneficial effects on the endothelium above its anti-hypertensive action. More work needs to be done in this area to ascertain whether these actions are translated to a longer-term prognostic benefit.

4.4.2. Potassium and Spironolactone

Potassium plays an important part in preserving the functional adequacy of the L-arginine-NO pathway. Taddei et al [172, 173] showed that intra-arterial administration of potassium chloride (KCL) significantly improved stimulated NO release in the forearm vasculature of hypertensive patients. Interestingly, there was no significant effect of KCL on agonist-evoked endothelial dependent vasodilation in the control normotensive group, suggesting an intriguing rule of potassium in NO bioactivity preservation in hypertension. The beneficial effect of potassium in hypertension has previously been highlighted; an analysis of the Syst-EUR trial has shown that hypokalaemia (<3.4mml/L) was associated with a higher incidence of cardiovascular events despite good BP control. Conversely, a high potassium diet appears to prevent deaths due to vascular strokes in hypertensive men, a disease also associated with endothelial dysfunction [174].

Spironolactone, a potassium-sparing diuretic with mineralocorticoid receptor antagonist has received much attention recently. It has been reported to improve NO bioactivity in patients with heart failure [175], consistent with the results of the RALES study in which the use of spironolactone reduced cardiac mortality by a third in subjects with grade III-IV heart failure [176]. The mechanism(s) by which aldosterone impairs endothelial function is unclear. Aldosterone it is known to enhance vascular responsiveness to pressor agents such as norepinephrine and angiotensin II even before the systemic blood pressure begins to increase

[177]. Also, aldosterone can cause direct vascular smooth muscle contraction via a non-genomic pathway that has not yet been characterised. In patients with secondary hypertension due to aldosterone producing adrenal adenomas, surgical excision of these tumours removed the excess circulating aldosterone resulting in a normalised acetylcholine vascular response, i.e. improved endothelial function and BP control [172].

Chronic treatment with aldosterone in rats has been shown to cause impairment of acetylcholine-induced relaxation and increased COX-2 expression in the endothelium of the thoracic aorta in rats [178], perhaps suggesting a mechanism for endothelial dysfunction caused by aldosterone. An interesting study by Garnier et al [179] examined 62 mice that were genetically modified to over-express aldosterone synthase (and thus over-produce aldosterone) and compared this group to normal mice. The authors found that although there was no difference in myocardial structure or cardiac function by echocardiography, there was a 55% decrease in basal coronary blood flow and vasodilatation to acetylcholine, bradykinin and sodium nitroprusside. Intriguingly, this suggests that there could be both NO-dependent and NO-independent mechanisms by which aldosterone mediates endothelial dysfunction. Given these findings, in theory, spironolactone or eplerenone should improve endothelial dysfunction in hypertensives where excess aldosterone is a factor and evidence has recently been obtained to suggest this.

Kobayashi et al [180] showed that eplerenone increased eNOS production and reduced oxidative stress and superoxide production in salt-sensitive rats with heart failure. A further study in salt sensitive rats found that the combination of eplerenone and amlodipine enhanced the improvement of vascular endothelial function, cardiac inflammation, fibrosis and diastolic dysfunction compared to that caused by amlodipine alone [181]. The improvement in endothelial function caused by eplerenone has also recently been found in humans [182]. Savoia et al [183] conducted a randomised controlled trial compared eplerenone to atenolol in 16 patients for 1 year and concluded that eplerenone treatment was associated with reduced arterial stiffness, decreased collagen/elastin ratio, and a reduction in circulating inflammatory mediators. The effects of eplerenone appear to be additive – as well as the combination with amlodipine described earlier, Imanishi et al [184] found a increased improvement in endothelial function using the combination of enalapril and aldosterone in rabbits.

The recent ESC guidelines for the management of heart failure [185] now place eplerenone and spironolactone as first line therapies – perhaps it is speculation, but the beneficial effects that have been noted in this group may be, at least in part, related to their beneficial effect on endothelial function.

4.4.3. Calcium Channel Blockers

Calcium channel blockers (CCBs) also have outcome data to support their use in hypertension. Two important studies, the NORDIL and INSIGHT trials have shown that diltiazem and long-acting nifedipine (GITS) respectively were as effective as thiazide diuretics in reducing cardiovascular mortality and morbidity in essential hypertension [186-188]. Calcium channel blockers have similarly been shown to have a beneficial effect on nitric oxide bioactivity in coronary, forearm and resistance (subcutaneous) vascular beds. In the forearm microcirculation, Lyons et al [188] have reported that 6-weeks treatment with amlodipine improved the vasoconstrictive response to L-NMMA (an inhibitor of eNOS) or basal NO release in newly diagnosed hypertensives. In a later study, Perticone et al [189] showed that oral isradipine also improved both stimulated (ACh-induced) and basal (L-

NMMA induced) NO release in hypertension. However, Taddei et al demonstrated contrasting effects on the endothelium with acute and chronic administration of a highly lipophilic calcium channel blocker, lacidipine [190]. This group showed that intra-arterial lacidipine did not significantly affect NO bioactivity, but chronic (2 and 8 months) oral treatment with this agent significantly improved stimulated NO release. Interestingly, the improved NO bioactivity persisted after 2-weeks of drug withdrawal, despite returning to hypertensive state. This suggests that BP control in itself may not be sufficient to improve NO release. In the majority of cases, hypertension is treated with combination therapy. Recently, a study by Yamamoto et al [191] found that azelnidpine in combination with olmesartan had improved endothelial function to a greater extent than olmesartan and hydrochlorothiazide.

Similar beneficial effects of calcium channel blockers on NO bioactivity have also been observed in smaller resistance vessels. The technique required for assessing endothelial function in these vessels involves gluteal subcutaneous tissue biopsy and myography. Schiffrin et al [192] have observed an improvement in acetylcholine (stimulated NO) response and vascular remodelling in these resistance vessels in hypertensives treated for 1 year with long acting nifedipine.

Of course, reversing endothelial dysfunction in the coronary arteries would be more relevant in hypertension if an improved cardiac outcome were the goal. Freielingsdolf et al [193] have shown that acute intracoronary administration of either nicardipine or diltiazem in hypertensives reversed endothelial dysfunction in both stenotic and non-stenotic epicardial coronary arteries. Of note, there was no significant effect on the endothelium (NO pathway) of these compounds in normal control subjects. The largest clinical trials looking at CCBs and endothelial function were the ENCORE studies [194, 195]. ENCORE I examined 343 patients undergoing percutaneous coronary intervention and randomised patients to patients were randomized in a double-blind manner to placebo, cerivastatin, nifedipine, or combination therapy for 6 months. In this study the authors demonstrated that nifedipine improved endothelial function at 6 months. In ENCORE II the authors were able to demonstrate that a controlled release preparation of nifedipine was able to improve endothelial function at 2 years.

Calcium channel blockers act directly on voltage dependent L-type calcium channels found on the vascular smooth muscle cells. Blockade of these channels reduces the influx of extracellular calcium into the sarcoplasmic reticulum facilitating vascular smooth muscle cell relaxation. However, endothelial cells are devoid of these receptors for calcium channel blockers to act on. Hence, the mechanism by which calcium channel blockers improve endothelial NO bioavailability is unclear. However, in the coronary microcirculation the addition of a calcium channel blocker appears to indirectly facilitate an increase in intracellular smooth muscle cell cGMP, which is the second messenger of NO and mediates its vasodilation. Therefore, as expected an increase in intracellular cGMP with calcium channel blockers enhances both endothelium dependent and independent vasodilation [193, 196]. This has been confirmed with both dihydropyridine and non-dihydropyridine calcium channel blockers. In contrast, in the forearm microcirculation, calcium channel blockers do not appear to influence the NO-independent pathway whenever exogenous organic sources of NO such as nitrates are present. Two additional mechanisms have been described to explain the effects of calcium channel blocker in the forearm circulation, which might be relevant to the coronary vasculature. The first explanation is that most calcium channel blockers have antioxidant activities [197, 198]. This reduces superoxide anions, which normally inactivate released NO hence reducing NO bioactivity. The second explanation involves a reduction in endothelin release by calcium channel blockers. Endothelin is a potent vasoconstrictor and it is released from the endothelium [199]. Normally, there is a balance between vasoconstrictive and vasodilating substances in the vasculature but in hypertension, the bioavailability of endothelin might be increased in parallel with a reduction in NO bioactivity. Kiowski et al [200, 201] have shown that calcium channel blockers contributed to improved NO bioactivity by reducing endothelin release. In addition, Cardillo et al [202] have recently shown that in patients with essential hypertension, the increased endothelin activity is partly responsible for the increased vascular tone [203]. Hence, in a model where vasoconstrictive activity is increased, such as hypertension, a reduction of endothelin release would improve NO bioactivity. Recently, another theory has also been postulated, that CCBs may reduce tissue plasminogen activator activity, thus reducing thrombogenic risk by decreasing platelet activation [204].

4.4.4. Angiotensin Converting Enzyme Inhibitors (ACE-I) and Angiotensin type 2 Receptor Blockers (ARBs)

Since the landmark study on renovascular hypertension by Goldblatt [205], it has been clear that the renin-angiotensin-aldosterone system (RAAS) plays an important role in BP regulation (figure 3). Angiotensin II stimulates angiotensin type 1 receptors (AT1) to mediate arteriolar vasoconstriction and remodelling, superoxide anion production, renal sodium reabsorption, aldosterone secretion and endothelin (ET-1) release [206]. Many of these actions affect the vascular endothelium adversely. On the other hand stimulation of the angiotensin type 2 (AT2) receptor by angiotensin has mainly opposing actions to those of AT1 stimulation and recently has been shown to contribute to endothelial NO release [207]. Hence, AT1 receptor blockade should eventually improve NO bioactivity.

AT2 production can be reduced by angiotensin converting enzyme inhibitors which also increase both tissue and plasma bradykinin by inhibiting kininase II [208]. By stimulating the B2 receptors, bradykinin mediates the release of NO, prostacyclin and the putative endothelial hyperpolarizing factor (EDHF); agents that produce vasodilation [209-211]. Two large studies have investigated the effects of ACE-I and ARBs in the coronary and forearm vasculature (TREND, BANFF) respectively in patients with atherosclerosis [212, 213]. The TREND study showed that quinapril reversed epicardial coronary artery endothelial dysfunction in patients with coronary artery disease. The BANFF study showed an improvement of endothelial dysfunction with quinapril, using reactive hyperaemia, in the forearm vasculature of patients with atherosclerosis. However, such a favourable effect of ACE-I on endothelial dysfunction is less consistent in hypertensives. Two independent long-term studies evaluating respectively the vascular responses to cilazapril and lisinopril on subcutaneous arteries (small resistance vessels) in essential hypertensives showed a considerable improvement in stimulated NO release following prolonged treatment with these agents [214, 215]. Similar results were obtained in the coronary microcirculation of hypertensive patients with ACE-I [216]. Antony et al showed that intravenous perindoprilat (the active metabolite of perindopril) restored the cold pressure test response and flow-mediated coronary artery vasodilation in 10 patients with untreated (newly diagnosed) essential hypertension. Taddei et al [217] have reported that 1 year of treatment with lisinopril improved endothelium-dependent and independent vasodilatation in forearm vasculature of hypertensives.

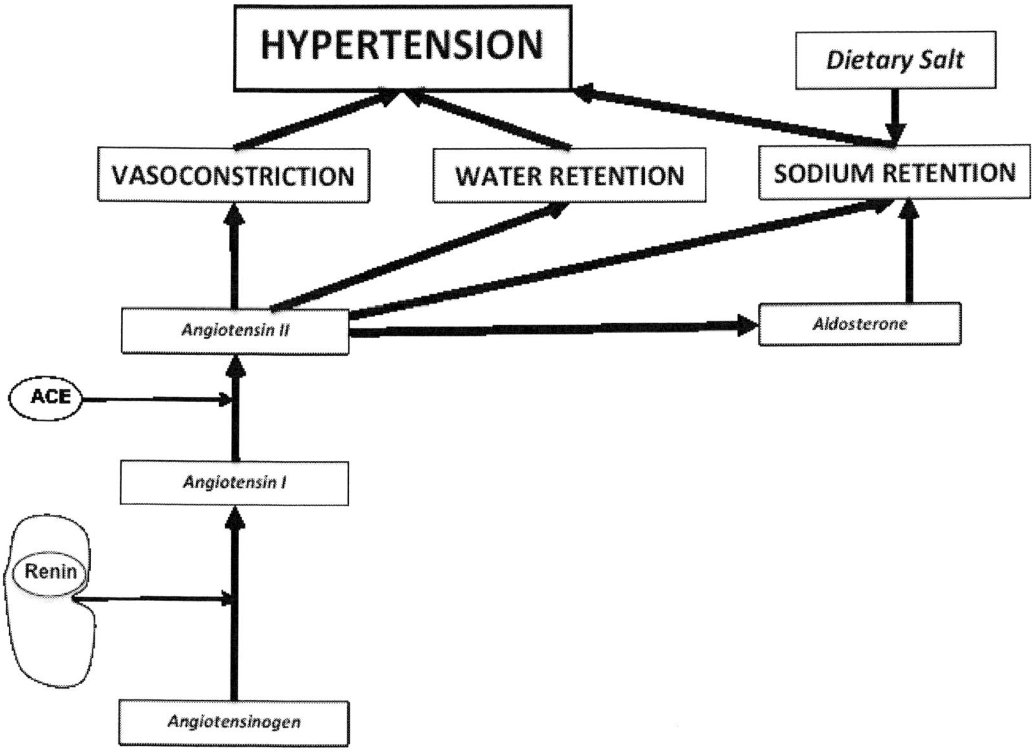

Figure 3. The renin-angiotensin-aldosterone system.

However, Kiowski et al [218] failed to find any improvement on NO bioactivity in the forearm vasculature after 5 months of oral cilazapril treatment despite adequate BP control in a group of hypertensives. Similarly, Creager et al [219] failed to improve NO bioactivity with 8 weeks treatment with either oral captopril or enalapril. However, two independent studies have shown an improvement of stimulated NO release following a single oral dose of captopril in such patients [220, 221]. Lyons et al [188] have investigated the effects of ACE-I on basal NO release in hypertensives. They showed that 6 weeks treatment with enalapril improved, but did not normalise, basal NO release in previously untreated hypertensives. Finally, in a large study involving 296 hypertensive patients, Higashi et al [153] using the technique of forearm reactive hyperaemia (flow-induced NO release) compared the endothelial vascular effects of calcium channel blockers, ACE-I, beta-blockers, and diuretics. They reported that only treatment with ACE-I significantly enhanced the forearm blood flow (an index of endothelium-dependent vasodilation) during reactive hyperaemia whilst the other drug classes had no significant effect although they did equally reduce blood pressure.

There are also reports of the beneficial effects of ARBs on the endothelial function. Schiffrin et al [152] reported that 1 of year treatment with losartan improved both functional and structural properties of small resistance (subcutaneous) arteries in hypertensive patients. Prasad et al [222] found the same in patients with atherosclerosis. In contrast, Ghiadoni et al [223] found that 1 year of treatment with candesartan improved stimulated NO release, but this was accompanied by a concomitant endothelium-independent improvement suggesting an alteration in vascular smooth muscle cell responsiveness. Tzemos et al [224] also found that valsartan mediated an improvement in endothelial function through both NO-dependent and independent pathways. Interestingly, amlodipine had no effect on nitric oxide. This was similar to the findings of Hirooka et al in large arteries [225].

In summary, blocking the renin-angiotensin-aldosterone system either at the conversion from Ang I to II or at the Ang II receptor level may favourably affect the NO bioactivity. It is likely that in the forearm microcirculation the tissue renin-angiotensin system is the predominant generator of Ang II hence only ACE-I with high tissue penetration (enough to block the tissue renin-angiotensin system) are likely to be effective [212, 226]. The two large studies, BANFF and TREND, might have obtained positive results because they involved quinalapril, a highly lipophilic ACE-I and this might explain the results. In a sub-analysis of the recent EUROPA study (examining the beneficial effects of ACE-inhibition in patients with stable coronary artery disease), perindopril appeared to increase expression and activity of eNOS by 19% and 27% respectively, as well as a significant reduction in plasma levels of angiotensin II, tumour necrosis factor-α and an increase in bradykinin, nitrate and nitrite [227].

All in all, although there are varying results in studies of ACEIs and ARBs, however the weight of evidence would tend to come down in favour of their beneficial effects. A recent meta-analysis by Miyamoto et al [228] found 38 studies looking at FMD with these two classes of drugs, and in the majority there was an improvement in endothelial function caused by ACEIs and ARBs. Recent studies have looked at the effects of angiotensin blockade in other subgroups, for example a study by Terashima et al [229] who found that telmisartan improved coronary endothelial function more than amlodipine in patients with drug eluting stents as measured by response to intracoronary infusion of acetylcholine.

Interestingly, a recent animal study [230] looked at the effects of aliskiren, a direct rennin inhibitor (the initial pathway of the renin-angiotensin-aldosterone axis). In this study, the authors found that aliskiren improved endothelial dysfunction in rat aortas and decreased oxidative stress. The effect of aliskiren was studied in humans by Virdis [231] in a comparative study against ramipril. Aliskiren produced a significantly greater reduction in augmentation index and improved the vasodilatory response to acetylcholine, however blood pressure and pulse wave reduction was the same in both groups. Meanwhile, Cherney et al suggest that direct renin inhibition using aliskiren might also provide better results than ACE inhibitors in type 2 diabetics [232]. These results may point to a slightly different action of aliskiren, and provide interesting directions for further research.

4.4.5. Endothelin Antagonists

Endothelin 1 (ET-1) acting through the ETA receptor is a potent vasoconstrictor that also promotes vascular smooth muscle cell proliferation [233, 234]. Its gene expression in the vessel wall is promoted by ATII, and its vasoconstrictive effect appears to be enhanced in hypertensives. It may thus play a role in the pathogenesis of hypertension [202, 235, 236]. However, the plasma levels of ET-1 have not been consistently found to be raised in hypertension [237, 238]. Nonetheless, ET-1 is released abluminally rather luminally, hence its plasma levels may not necessarily reflect its activity [239]. Increased ET-1 activity has been found in salt-sensitive hypertension [240, 241]. In animal models of hypertension ET-1 blockade significantly reduces BP and prevents the development of target organ damage

[151]. In human hypertension, Cardillo et al have shown that forearm intrabrachial administration of both selective and non-selective endothelin receptor blockers improved endothelium-dependent vasodilation. The vasodilating properties of endothelin-1 receptor blockers might explain the beneficial effects on BP of bosentan, a non-selective ET-1 receptor blocker. Krum et al [242] have shown that 4 weeks of treatment with bosentan reduced blood pressure as effectively as enalapril. Moreover, the favourable effect of treatment with bosentan on blood pressure occurred without reflexive neurohormonal activation, which may suggest a more targeted effect of this drug on endothelial ET-1. Coronary endothelial function has also been shown to be improved by atrasentan [243]. A synergistic effect with phosphodiesterase type 5 inhibitors has also been recently found in rats [244].

A recent study has investigated the effects of relaxin on aortic stiffness in rats. Relaxin is a member of the insulin superfamily and has effects on NO production. It also acts as an endothelin receptor antagonist [245, 246]. Acetylcholine mediated endothelial function improved following infusion of relaxin in these rats. The authors noted no difference in eNOS expression but there was increased eNOS activity. Superoxide production was also decreased. Perhaps relaxin may provide a novel target for treatment of endothelial dysfunction.

4.4.6. Vasopeptidase Inhibitors

Vasopeptidase inhibition is a relatively novel concept in blood pressure regulation and in cardiovascular medicine [247]. The actions of this new class of drugs involve the simultaneous inhibition of two different enzymes: angiotensin converting enzyme (ACE) and neutral endopeptidase (NEP). Neutral endopeptidase which degrades natriuretic peptides is widely distributed in endothelial cells, cardiac myocytes, vascular smooth muscle cells and renal epithelial cells [248]. The natriuretic peptides (ANP, BNP, CNP) play a prominent role in cardio-renal blood pressure homeostasis and also in vascular tone and structure [249, 250]. Omapatrilat, a vasopeptidase inhibitor under development, reduces blood pressure more efficiently compared to ACE-I [251]. In theory the dual action of omapatrilat on the NEP/ACE should produce a more substantial vascular response than single enzyme inhibition. This is particularly true in clinical settings where natriuretic peptides are activated, such as salt-sensitive hypertension or in high-renin hypertension. [252, 253]. In 2001, d'Uscio et al showed that omapatrilat prevented endothelial dysfunction in resistance arteries of salt-sensitive rats. Importantly, in the same study omapatrilat better preserved both structural and functional properties of the arterial wall than captopril. These effects are also seen in the renal vasculature [254]. While there have been several further studies showing a beneficial effect in animals, including in combination with angiotensin blockade [255, 256], there is still yet to be a large study in humans.

4.5. Antioxidants

Impairment in NO bioactivity may be secondary to either decreased synthesis-release and/or increased NO inactivation. Nitric oxide (an anion), after synthesis, is rapidly inactivated by locally (of endothelial and extra-endothelial origin) generated oxygen-derived free radicals ($O^{-}2$) to form peroxynitrite anions ($OONO^{-}$), which have considerably less vasodilating capacity than NO [57, 58]. The chemical reaction between NO and superoxide anions is extremely fast, faster than that with superoxide dismutase (SODs) or with plasma vitamins which are natural scavengers of superoxide anions. An increase in free-radical formation otherwise known as oxidative stress is present in many cardiovascular diseases including hypertension, hyperlipidaemia and heart failure [59-62]. Interestingly, the severity of hypertension appears to correlate with the degree of underlying oxidative stress [63]. Antioxidants, whether endogenous or exogenous in origin are part of an additional scavenging mechanism directed to "overcome" the excess of superoxide anion production. Hypertension has been described as a disease characterised by an excess of oxygen free radicals coupled with an inefficient antioxidant mechanism [61, 64, 65]. There is evidence to suggest that hypertensive patients have significantly lower plasma concentrations of naturally occurring antioxidant factors (thiols, vitamins A, C, E) compared with matched normotensive volunteers. Also free radical scavengers such as superoxide dismutase (SOD), and glutathione (GSH) are reported to be depressed in hypertensive patients [66, 67]. Taddei et al [257] reported that intra-brachial (forearm) administration of vitamin C, a potent antioxidant, improved both stimulated and basal NO release in hypertensive patients [258] and this has been confirmed by others [61]. Similar effects of vitamin C on NO bioactivity were also obtained in the coronary circulation of hypertensive patients after the intracoronary administration of vitamin C [259]. Also, Jeserich et al [260], using the cold pressor testing showed an improvement of endothelial dysfunction in the epicardial coronary arteries of patients with hypertension following infusion of vitamin C. Improved endothelial function has also been shown by Engler et al in children with hyperlipidaemia treated with vitamins C and E [261].

The effect of chronic oral vitamin C on BP lowering has been less consistent. The available data are conflicting with some investigators finding a positive effect whilst others do not [262-265]. The dosages of vitamin C involved in these studies varied widely from 400 to 2000mg daily. Duffy et al [264] reported that regular vitamin C supplementation (1 gram daily) reduced blood pressure but this was unrelated to endothelial dysfunction. The studies which showed an improvement in endothelial dysfunction in hypertension all used intra-arterially administered vitamin C where it achieved very high or supra-physiological plasma concentrations. Indeed, because of the nature of the pharmacokinetics between NO and superoxide radicals, high plasma levels of any antioxidants would have been necessary to maintain a constant and effective scavenging system. Sherman et al recently addressed this issue. They showed that, at least in the forearm microcirculation following intra-arterial infusions of vitamin C, its plasma concentration was the main determinant of achieving endothelium-dependent vasodilation and that lower concentrations of vitamin C failed to exert any biological effect. However, recent conflicting evidence has been published suggesting that at least in elderly patients, administration of vitamin C can acute reverse endothelial dysfunction [266]. This effect was not seen in younger patients in this study, and perhaps suggests that the beneficial effects of anti-oxidants and the mechanism by which oxidative stress causes endothelial dysfunction is perhaps age-related.

Not all antioxidants have been shown to be equally effective in reversing endothelial dysfunction. Garcia et al [267] reported that copper-zinc dismutase, another endothelial superoxide scavenger, did not have a significant effect on acetylcholine-induced endothelial-dependent vasodilation in hypertensive patients. Of note is the fact that in contrast to the high intracellular penetration of vitamin C, copper-zinc dismutase, which is negatively charged, is unable to penetrate the cells. Hence, the use of copper-zinc superoxide dismutase assesses and buffers only the extracellular oxidative environment rather than the intracellular or intimal space. Interestingly, in animal studies the beneficial effects of copper-zinc superoxide dismutase were only obtained after modification of the enzyme to gain access to the endothelial surface [61, 268]. Assessing another antioxidant, Panza et al [269] failed to show any benefit on the NO pathway by using oxypurinol, an inhibitor of xanthine-oxidase. Although superoxide radicals have been implicated in the genesis and perpetuation of cardiovascular diseases [64], and there is an association between hypertension and increased oxidative stress, the benefits of therapeutic interventions directed to reduce oxidative stress are not evident [270]. Of course, not all anti-oxidants are equal, and so there is still potential for this class of drug to become therapeutically useful.

Conclusion

Endothelial dysfunction is associated with hypertension and its presence correlates with target organ damage. Furthermore, endothelial dysfunction may be both a cause and a consequence of hypertension. In this chapter, we have discussed the pathways by which endothelial dysfunction may occur and the clinical evidence of its utility. Finally, we discussed the evidence looking at reversal of endothelial function, both by antihypertensive medications and therapies more directly targeted at the endothelium. Antihypertensive drug treatment improves and in some cases reverses endothelial dysfunction but this appear to depend very much on drug class and the vascular territories studied. Although calcium channel blockers, ACE-I, and ARBs seem to outperform beta-blockers (with the exception of nebivolol) and diuretics in terms of improving endothelial dysfunction, they do not seem to produce a greater antihypertensive effect. Most importantly, there is still some doubt within the scientific community as to whether the improvement in endothelial function is translated into long-term prognostic benefit. Interestingly the most effective strategy by far to improve endothelial dysfunction is regular aerobic exercise although its antihypertensive effect is only modest and less than most antihypertensive drugs. Recently proposed targets for endothelial dysfunction include oestrogens [271, 272], sirtuins (proteins possessing either histone deacetylase or mono-ribosyltransferase activity) [273] and the effects of coronary stents of endothelial function [274, 275]. Perhaps the most important future direction in this field however is the accumulation of prognostic data regarding endothelial function, especially in various conditions, for example heart failure [276].

Therefore, although endothelial dysfunction is a conceptually attractive therapeutic target in hypertension, at this point in time, we lack convincing data that using endothelial dysfunction to guide our treatment would produce any better outcomes than using blood pressure targets to guide our treatment. This situation may change in the near future as more trials are conducted in this fascinating area.

References

[1] Furchgott, R.F. and J.V. Zawadzki, The obligatory role of endothelial cells in the relaxation of arterial smooth muscle by acetylcholine. *Nature*, 1980. 288(5789): p. 373-6.

[2] Henry, Y., et al., EPR characterization of molecular targets for NO in mammalian cells and organelles. *FASEB J,* 1993. 7(12): p. 1124-34.

[3] Moncada, S. and A. Higgs, The L-arginine-nitric oxide pathway. *N Engl J Med*, 1993. 329(27): p. 2002-12.

[4] Calver, A., J. Collier, and P. Vallance, Nitric oxide and cardiovascular control. *Exp Physiol*, 1993. 78(3): p. 303-26.

[5] Vallance, P., J. Collier, and S. Moncada, Effects of endothelium-derived nitric oxide on peripheral arteriolar tone in man. *Lancet*, 1989. 2(8670): p. 997-1000.

[6] Hibbs, J.B., Jr., R.R. Taintor, and Z. Vavrin, Macrophage cytotoxicity: role for L-arginine deiminase and imino nitrogen oxidation to nitrite. *Science*, 1987. 235(4787): p. 473-6.

[7] Amezcua, J.L., et al., Nitric oxide synthesized from L-arginine regulates vascular tone in the coronary circulation of the rabbit. *Br J Pharmacol*, 1989. 97(4): p. 1119-24.

[8] Furchgott, R.F., Role of endothelium in responses of vascular smooth muscle. *Circ Res*, 1983. 53(5): p. 557-73.

[9] Gorog, P. and I.B. Kovacs, Inhibition of vascular smooth muscle cell migration by intact endothelium is nitric oxide-mediated: interference by oxidised low density lipoproteins. *J Vasc Res*, 1998. 35(3): p. 165-9.

[10] Tare, M., et al., Hyperpolarization and relaxation of arterial smooth muscle caused by nitric oxide derived from the endothelium. *Nature*, 1990. 346(6279): p. 69-71.

[11] Kanwar, S. and P. Kubes, Nitric oxide is an antiadhesive molecule for leukocytes. *New Horiz*, 1995. 3(1): p. 93-104.

[12] Radomski, M.W. and S. Moncada, Regulation of vascular homeostasis by nitric oxide. *Thromb Haemost,* 1993. 70(1): p. 36-41.

[13] Wennmalm, A., et al., Metabolism and excretion of nitric oxide in humans. An experimental and clinical study. Circ Res, 1993. 73(6): p. 1121-7.

[14] Rubanyi, G.M., et al., Mechanoreception by the endothelium: mediators and mechanisms of pressure- and flow-induced vascular responses. *Blood Vessels*, 1990. 27(2-5): p. 246-57.

[15] Pohl, U., et al., Crucial role of endothelium in the vasodilator response to increased flow in vivo. *Hypertension*, 1986. 8(1): p. 37-44.

[16] Rees, D.D., et al., A specific inhibitor of nitric oxide formation from L-arginine attenuates endothelium-dependent relaxation. *Br J Pharmacol*, 1989. 96(2): p. 418-24.

[17] Haynes, W.G., et al., Inhibition of nitric oxide synthesis increases blood pressure in healthy humans. *J Hypertens*, 1993. 11(12): p. 1375-80.

[18] Bech, J.N., et al., Dietary sodium affects systemic and renal hemodynamic response to NO inhibition in healthy humans. *Am J Physiol*, 1998. 274(5 Pt 2): p. F914-23.

[19] Anggard, E., Nitric oxide: mediator, murderer, and medicine. *Lancet*, 1994. 343(8907): p. 1199-206.

[20] Luscher, T.F. and P.M. Vanhoutte, Endothelium-dependent contractions to acetylcholine in the aorta of the spontaneously hypertensive rat. *Hypertension*, 1986. 8(4): p. 344-8.

[21] Rand, M.J., Nitrergic transmission: nitric oxide as a mediator of non-adrenergic, non-cholinergic neuro-effector transmission. *Clin Exp Pharmacol Physiol*, 1992. 19(3): p. 147-69.

[22] Toda, N. and T. Okamura, Role of nitric oxide in neurally induced cerebroarterial relaxation. *J Pharmacol Exp Ther,* 1991. 258(3): p. 1027-32.
[23] Chowdhary, S. and J.N. Townend, Role of nitric oxide in the regulation of cardiovascular autonomic control. *Clin Sci (Lond),* 1999. 97(1): p. 5-17.
[24] Luscher, T.F., Imbalance of endothelium-derived relaxing and contracting factors. A new concept in hypertension? *Am J Hypertens*, 1990. 3(4): p. 317-30.
[25] Levy, D., et al., Prognostic implications of echocardiographically determined left ventricular mass in the Framingham Heart Study. *N Engl J Med,* 1990. 322(22): p. 1561-6.
[26] Heagerty, A.M., et al., Small artery structure in hypertension. Dual processes of remodeling and growth. *Hypertension*, 1993. 21(4): p. 391-7.
[27] Dilley, R.J., et al., Vascular hypertrophy in renal hypertensive spontaneously hypertensive rats. Hypertension, 1994. 24(1): p. 8-15.
[28] Mulvany, M.J., The fourth Sir George Pickering memorial lecture. The structure of the resistance vasculature in essential hypertension. *J Hypertens*, 1987. 5(2): p. 129-36.
[29] Kamiya, A. and T. Togawa, Adaptive regulation of wall shear stress to flow change in the canine carotid artery. *Am J Physiol,* 1980. 239(1): p. H14-21.
[30] Guyton, J.R. and C.J. Hartley, Flow restriction of one carotid artery in juvenile rats inhibits growth of arterial diameter. *Am J Physiol,* 1985. 248(4 Pt 2): p. H540-6.
[31] Langille, B.L. and F. O'Donnell, Reductions in arterial diameter produced by chronic decreases in blood flow are endothelium-dependent. *Science*, 1986. 231(4736): p. 405-7.
[32] Olivetti, G., et al., Morphometry of medial hypertrophy in the rat thoracic aorta. *Lab Invest*, 1980. 42(5): p. 559-65.
[33] Harder, D.R., Pressure-induced myogenic activation of cat cerebral arteries is dependent on intact endothelium. *Circ Res,* 1987. 60(1): p. 102-7.
[34] Iba, T., et al., Stimulation of endothelial secretion of tissue-type plasminogen activator by repetitive stretch. *J Surg Re*s, 1991. 50(5): p. 457-60.
[35] Ranieri, G., et al., The effects of diuretic and beta-blocker treatment on cardiac and vascular structural changes in untreated essential hypertensive patients. J *Hypertens Suppl*, 1993. 11(5): p. S368-9.
[36] Morishita, R., et al., Possible role of the vascular renin-angiotensin system in hypertension and vascular hypertrophy. *Hypertension*, 1992. 19(2 Suppl): p. II62-7.
[37] Iwatsuki, K., et al., Hypertension: increase of collagen biosynthesis in arteries but not in veins. *Science*, 1977. 198(4315): p. 403-5.
[38] Dzau, V.J. and G.H. Gibbons, Endothelium and growth factors in vascular remodeling of hypertension. *Hypertension*, 1991. 18(5 Suppl): p. III115-21.
[39] Luscher, T.F., L. Raij, and P.M. Vanhoutte, Endothelium-dependent vascular responses in normotensive and hypertensive Dahl rats. *Hypertension*, 1987. 9(2): p. 157-63.
[40] Raij, L., T.F. Luscher, and P.M. Vanhoutte, High potassium diet augments endothelium-dependent relaxations in the Dahl rat. *Hypertension*, 1988. 12(6): p. 562-7.
[41] Konishi, M. and C. Su, Role of endothelium in dilator responses of spontaneously hypertensive rat arteries. *Hypertension*, 1983. 5(6): p. 881-6.
[42] Winquist, R.J., et al., Decreased endothelium-dependent relaxation in New Zealand genetic hypertensive rats. *J Hypertens,* 1984. 2(5): p. 541-5.

[43] Lockette, W., Y. Otsuka, and O. Carretero, The loss of endothelium-dependent vascular relaxation in hypertension. *Hypertension*, 1986. 8(6 Pt 2): p. II61-6.

[44] Luscher, T.F., P.M. Vanhoutte, and L. Raij, Antihypertensive treatment normalizes decreased endothelium-dependent relaxations in rats with salt-induced hypertension. *Hypertension*, 1987. 9(6 Pt 2): p. III193-7.

[45] Luscher, T.F., Endothelium-derived vasoactive factors and regulation of vascular tone in human blood vessels. *Lung*, 1990. 168 Suppl: p. 27-34.

[46] Luscher, T.F., et al., Endothelium-derived contracting factors. *Hypertension*, 1992. 19(2): p. 117-30.

[47] Panza, J.A., et al., Abnormal endothelium-dependent vascular relaxation in patients with essential hypertension. *N Engl J Med,* 1990. 323(1): p. 22-7.

[48] Panza, J.A., Endothelium-dependent vasodilatation and essential hypertension. *N Engl J Med,* 1994. 331(14): p. 951.

[49] Calver, A., J. Collier, and P. Vallance, Forearm blood flow responses to a nitric oxide synthase inhibitor in patients with treated essential hypertension. *Cardiovasc Res*, 1994. 28(11): p. 1720-5.

[50] Calver, A., et al., Effect of local intra-arterial NG-monomethyl-L-arginine in patients with hypertension: the nitric oxide dilator mechanism appears abnormal. *J Hypertens*, 1992. 10(9): p. 1025-31.

[51] Panza, J.A., et al., Role of endothelium-derived nitric oxide in the abnormal endothelium-dependent vascular relaxation of patients with essential hypertension. *Circulation*, 1993. 87(5): p. 1468-74.

[52] Cockcroft, J.R., et al., Preserved endothelium-dependent vasodilatation in patients with essential hypertension. *N Engl J Med,* 1994. 330(15): p. 1036-40.

[53] Bruning, T.A., et al., In vivo characterization of muscarinic receptor subtypes that mediate vasodilatation in patients with essential hypertension. *Hypertension*, 1995. 26(1): p. 70-7.

[54] Touyz, R.M., Reactive oxygen species, vascular oxidative stress, and redox signaling in hypertension: what is the clinical significance? *Hypertension*, 2004. 44(3): p. 248-52.

[55] Lip, G.Y., et al., Oxidative stress in malignant and non-malignant phase hypertension. *J Hum Hypertens*, 2002. 16(5): p. 333-6.

[56] Higashi, Y., et al., Endothelial function and oxidative stress in renovascular hypertension. *N Engl J Med,* 2002. 346(25): p. 1954-62.

[57] Beckman, J.S., et al., Apparent hydroxyl radical production by peroxynitrite: implications for endothelial injury from nitric oxide and superoxide. *Proc Natl Acad Sci U S A*, 1990. 87(4): p. 1620-4.

[58] Rubanyi, G.M. and P.M. Vanhoutte, Superoxide anions and hyperoxia inactivate endothelium-derived relaxing factor. *Am J Physiol*, 1986. 250(5 Pt 2): p. H822-7.

[59] Laursen, J.B., et al., Role of superoxide in angiotensin II-induced but not catecholamine-induced hypertension. *Circulation*, 1997. 95(3): p. 588-93.

[60] Rajagopalan, S., et al., Angiotensin II-mediated hypertension in the rat increases vascular superoxide production via membrane NADH/NADPH oxidase activation. Contribution to alterations of vasomotor tone. *J Clin Invest,* 1996. 97(8): p. 1916-23.

[61] Sherman, D.L., et al., Pharmacological concentrations of ascorbic acid are required for the beneficial effect on endothelial vasomotor function in hypertension. *Hypertension*, 2000. 35(4): p. 936-41.

[62] Prabha, P.S., et al., Free radical generation, lipid peroxidation and essential fatty acids in uncontrolled essential hypertension. *Prostaglandins Leukot Essent Fatty Acids,* 1990. 41(1): p. 27-33.

[63] Pierdomenico, S.D., et al., Blunted nocturnal fall in blood pressure and oxidative stress in men and women with essential hypertension. *Am J Hypertens*, 1999. 12(4 Pt 1): p. 356-63.

[64] Halliwell, B., Free radicals, antioxidants, and human disease: curiosity, cause, or consequence? *Lancet*, 1994. 344(8924): p. 721-4.

[65] Tse, W.Y., et al., Antioxidant status in controlled and uncontrolled hypertension and its relationship to endothelial damage. *J Hum Hypertens*, 1994. 8(11): p. 843-9.

[66] Sagar, S., et al., Oxygen free radicals in essential hypertension. *Mol Cell Biochem*, 1992. 111(1-2): p. 103-8.

[67] Dhalla, N.S., R.M. Temsah, and T. Netticadan, Role of oxidative stress in cardiovascular diseases. *J Hypertens*, 2000. 18(6): p. 655-73.

[68] Benzuly, K.H., et al., Functional improvement precedes structural regression of atherosclerosis. *Circulation*, 1994. 89(4): p. 1810-8.

[69] Brush, J.E., Jr., et al., Angina due to coronary microvascular disease in hypertensive patients without left ventricular hypertrophy. *N Engl J Med*, 1988. 319(20): p. 1302-7.

[70] Treasure, C.B., et al., Epicardial coronary artery responses to acetylcholine are impaired in hypertensive patients. *Circ Res*, 1992. 71(4): p. 776-81.

[71] Egashira, K., et al., Impaired coronary blood flow response to acetylcholine in patients with coronary risk factors and proximal atherosclerotic lesions. *J Clin Invest*, 1993. 91(1): p. 29-37.

[72] Egashira, K., et al., Impaired endothelium-dependent vasodilation of large epicardial and resistance coronary arteries in patients with essential hypertension. Different responses to acetylcholine and substance P. *Hypertension*, 1995. 25(2): p. 201-6.

[73] Quyyumi, A.A., et al., Endothelial dysfunction in patients with chest pain and normal coronary arteries. *Circulation*, 1992. 86(6): p. 1864-71.

[74] Bhagat, K., Endothelial function and myocardial infarction. *Cardiovasc Res*, 1998. 39(2): p. 312-7.

[75] Ghiadoni, L., et al., Endothelial function and common carotid artery wall thickening in patients with essential hypertension. *Hypertension*, 1998. 32(1): p. 25-32.

[76] Poli, A., et al., Ultrasonographic measurement of the common carotid artery wall thickness in hypercholesterolemic patients. A new model for the quantitation and follow-up of preclinical atherosclerosis in living human subjects. *Atherosclerosis*, 1988. 70(3): p. 253-61.

[77] Salonen, J.T. and R. Salonen, Ultrasonographically assessed carotid morphology and the risk of coronary heart disease. *Arterioscler Thromb*, 1991. 11(5): p. 1245-9.

[78] Devereux, R.B. and M.H. Alderman, Role of preclinical cardiovascular disease in the evolution from risk factor exposure to development of morbid events. *Circulation*, 1993. 88(4 Pt 1): p. 1444-55.

[79] Koren, M.J., et al., Relation of left ventricular mass and geometry to morbidity and mortality in uncomplicated essential hypertension. *Ann Intern Med,* 1991. 114(5): p. 345-52.

[80] Bikkina, M., et al., Left ventricular mass and risk of stroke in an elderly cohort. The Framingham Heart Study. *JAMA*, 1994. 272(1): p. 33-6.

[81] Roman, M.J., et al., Parallel cardiac and vascular adaptation in hypertension. *Circulation*, 1992. 86(6): p. 1909-18.

[82] Roman, M.J., et al., Relation of arterial structure and function to left ventricular geometric patterns in hypertensive adults. *J Am Coll Cardiol*, 1996. 28(3): p. 751-6.

[83] Roman, M.J., et al., Association of carotid atherosclerosis and left ventricular hypertrophy. *J Am Coll Cardiol,* 1995. 25(1): p. 83-90.

[84] Perticone, F., et al., Relationship between left ventricular mass and endothelium-dependent vasodilation in never-treated hypertensive patients. *Circulation*, 1999. 99(15): p. 1991-6.

[85] Millgard, J., et al., Left ventricular hypertrophy is associated with an attenuated endothelium-dependent vasodilation in hypertensive men. *Blood Press,* 2000. 9(6): p. 309-14.

[86] von zur Muhlen, B., et al., Ambulatory blood pressure and endothelium-dependent vasodilation in hypertensive patients. *Blood Press*, 2000. 9(2-3): p. 110-5.

[87] Forte, P., et al., Basal nitric oxide synthesis in essential hypertension. *Lancet*, 1997. 349(9055): p. 837-42.

[88] Gerhard, M., et al., Aging progressively impairs endothelium-dependent vasodilation in forearm resistance vessels of humans. *Hypertension*, 1996. 27(4): p. 849-53.

[89] Celermajer, D.S., et al., Endothelium-dependent dilation in the systemic arteries of asymptomatic subjects relates to coronary risk factors and their interaction. *J Am Coll Cardiol,* 1994. 24(6): p. 1468-74.

[90] Suwaidi, J.A., et al., Long-term follow-up of patients with mild coronary artery disease and endothelial dysfunction. *Circulation*, 2000. 101(9): p. 948-54.

[91] Halcox, J.P., et al., Prognostic value of coronary vascular endothelial dysfunction. *Circulation*, 2002. 106(6): p. 653-8.

[92] Schachinger, V. and A.M. Zeiher, Atherosclerosis-associated endothelial dysfunction. Z Kardiol, 2000. 89 Suppl 9: p. IX/70-4.

[93] Heitzer, T., et al., Endothelial dysfunction, oxidative stress, and risk of cardiovascular events in patients with coronary artery disease. *Circulation*, 2001. 104(22): p. 2673-8.

[94] Neunteufl, T., et al., Late prognostic value of flow-mediated dilation in the brachial artery of patients with chest pain. *Am J Cardiol,* 2000. 86(2): p. 207-10.

[95] Yeboah, J., et al., Brachial flow-mediated dilation predicts incident cardiovascular events in older adults: the Cardiovascular Health Study. *Circulation*, 2007. 115(18): p. 2390-7.

[96] Perticone, F., et al., Prognostic significance of endothelial dysfunction in hypertensive patients. *Circulation*, 2001. 104(2): p. 191-6.

[97] Modena, M.G., et al., Prognostic role of reversible endothelial dysfunction in hypertensive postmenopausal women. *J Am Coll Cardiol*, 2002. 40(3): p. 505-10.

[98] Anderson, T.J., et al., Microvascular function predicts cardiovascular events in primary prevention: long-term results from the Firefighters and Their Endothelium (FATE) study. *Circulation*, 2011. 123(2): p. 163-9.

[99] Philpott, A.C., et al., Comparison of new measures of vascular function to flow mediated dilatation as a measure of cardiovascular risk factors. *Am J Cardiol*, 2009. 103(11): p. 1610-5.

[100] Andersson, O.K., et al., Survival in treated hypertension: follow up study after two decades. *BMJ*, 1998. 317(7152): p. 167-71.

[101] Vallance, P., *Hypertension*. J R Coll Physicians Lond, 1999. 33(2): p. 119-23.
[102] Kokkinos, P.F., et al., Effects of regular exercise on blood pressure and left ventricular hypertrophy in African-American men with severe hypertension. *N Engl J Med*, 1995. 333(22): p. 1462-7.
[103] Duncan, J.J., et al., The effects of aerobic exercise on plasma catecholamines and blood pressure in patients with mild essential hypertension. *JAMA*, 1985. 254(18): p. 2609-13.
[104] Ramsay, L.E., et al., British Hypertension Society guidelines for hypertension management 1999: summary. *BMJ*, 1999. 319(7210): p. 630-5.
[105] Green, D.J., et al., Modification of forearm resistance vessels by exercise training in young men. *J Appl Physiol*, 1994. 77(4): p. 1829-33.
[106] Higashi, Y., et al., Regular aerobic exercise augments endothelium-dependent vascular relaxation in normotensive as well as hypertensive subjects: role of endothelium-derived nitric oxide. *Circulation*, 1999. 100(11): p. 1194-202.
[107] Taddei, S., et al., Aging and endothelial function in normotensive subjects and patients with essential hypertension. *Circulation*, 1995. 91(7): p. 1981-7.
[108] Kugiyama, K., et al., Impairment of endothelium-dependent arterial relaxation by lysolecithin in modified low-density lipoproteins. *Nature*, 1990. 344(6262): p. 160-2.
[109] Chin, J.H., S. Azhar, and B.B. Hoffman, Inactivation of endothelial derived relaxing factor by oxidized lipoproteins. *J Clin Invest*, 1992. 89(1): p. 10-8.
[110] Hambrecht, R., et al., Effect of exercise on coronary endothelial function in patients with coronary artery disease. *N Engl J Med,* 2000. 342(7): p. 454-60.
[111] Cornelissen, V.A., et al., Exercise-based cardiac rehabiliation improves endothelial function assessed by flow-mediated dilation but not by pulse amplitude tonometry. *Eur J Prev Cardiol*, 2012.
[112] Pasceri, V., J.T. Willerson, and E.T. Yeh, Direct proinflammatory effect of C-reactive protein on human endothelial cells. *Circulation*, 2000. 102(18): p. 2165-8.
[113] Ridker, P.M., et al., Comparison of C-reactive protein and low-density lipoprotein cholesterol levels in the prediction of first cardiovascular events. *N Engl J Med*, 2002. 347(20): p. 1557-65.
[114] Milani, R.V., C.J. Lavie, and M.R. Mehra, Reduction in C-reactive protein through cardiac rehabilitation and exercise training. *J Am Coll Cardiol*, 2004. 43(6): p. 1056-61.
[115] Vona, M., et al., Effects of different types of exercise training followed by detraining on endothelium-dependent dilation in patients with recent myocardial infarction. *Circulation*, 2009. 119(12): p. 1601-8.
[116] Vita, J.A., et al., Coronary vasomotor response to acetylcholine relates to risk factors for coronary artery disease. *Circulation*, 1990. 81(2): p. 491-7.
[117] Taddei, S., et al., Hypertension causes premature aging of endothelial function in humans. *Hypertension*, 1997. 29(3): p. 736-43.
[118] Al-Shaer, M.H., et al., Effects of aging and atherosclerosis on endothelial and vascular smooth muscle function in humans. *Int J Cardiol*, 2006. 109(2): p. 201-6.
[119] Herrera, M.D., et al., Endothelial dysfunction and aging: an update. *Ageing Res Rev*, 2010. 9(2): p. 142-52.
[120] Erusalimsky, J.D. and C. Skene, Mechanisms of endothelial senescence. *Exp Physiol*, 2009. 94(3): p. 299-304.
[121] Casino, P.R., et al., The role of nitric oxide in endothelium-dependent vasodilation of hypercholesterolemic patients. *Circulation*, 1993. 88(6): p. 2541-7.

[122] Creager, M.A., et al., Impaired vasodilation of forearm resistance vessels in hypercholesterolemic humans. *J Clin Invest,* 1990. 86(1): p. 228-34.
[123] Vogel, R.A., M.C. Corretti, and G.D. Plotnick, Effect of a single high-fat meal on endothelial function in healthy subjects. *Am J Cardiol*, 1997. 79(3): p. 350-4.
[124] Steinberg, H.O., et al., Endothelial dysfunction is associated with cholesterol levels in the high normal range in humans. *Circulation*, 1997. 96(10): p. 3287-93.
[125] Muiesan, M.L., et al., Effect of treatment on flow-dependent vasodilation of the brachial artery in essential hypertension. Hypertension, 1999. 33(1 Pt 2): p. 575-80.
[126] Okumura, K., et al., Small Low-Density Lipoprotein Cholesterol Concentration is a Determinant of Endothelial Dysfunction by Peripheral Artery Tonometry in Men. J Atheroscler Thromb, 2012.
[127] Ashen, M.D. and R.S. Blumenthal, Clinical practice. Low HDL cholesterol levels. *N Engl J Med*, 2005. 353(12): p. 1252-60.
[128] Barter, P., et al., HDL cholesterol, very low levels of LDL cholesterol, and cardiovascular events. *N Engl J Med*, 2007. 357(13): p. 1301-10.
[129] Bisoendial, R.J., et al., Restoration of endothelial function by increasing high-density lipoprotein in subjects with isolated low high-density lipoprotein. *Circulation*, 2003. 107(23): p. 2944-8.
[130] Spieker, L.E., et al., High-density lipoprotein restores endothelial function in hypercholesterolemic men. *Circulation*, 2002. 105(12): p. 1399-402.
[131] Nicholls, S.J., et al., Reconstituted high-density lipoproteins inhibit the acute pro-oxidant and proinflammatory vascular changes induced by a periarterial collar in normocholesterolemic rabbits. *Circulation*, 2005. 111(12): p. 1543-50.
[132] Sorrentino, S.A., et al., Endothelial-vasoprotective effects of high-density lipoprotein are impaired in patients with type 2 diabetes mellitus but are improved after extended-release niacin therapy. *Circulation*, 2010. 121(1): p. 110-22.
[133] McVeigh, G.E., et al., Effects of long-term cigarette smoking on endothelium-dependent responses in humans. *Am J Cardiol,* 1996. 78(6): p. 668-72.
[134] Celermajer, D.S., et al., Cigarette smoking is associated with dose-related and potentially reversible impairment of endothelium-dependent dilation in healthy young adults. *Circulation*, 1993. 88(5 Pt 1): p. 2149-55.
[135] Toda, N. and H. Toda, Nitric oxide-mediated blood flow regulation as affected by smoking and nicotine. *Eur J Pharmacol,* 2010. 649(1-3): p. 1-13.
[136] Bermudez, E.A., et al., Relation between markers of systemic vascular inflammation and smoking in women. *Am J Cardiol*, 2002. 89(9): p. 1117-9.
[137] Mendall, M.A., et al., Relation of serum cytokine concentrations to cardiovascular risk factors and coronary heart disease. *Heart*, 1997. 78(3): p. 273-7.
[138] Taddei, S., et al., Menopause is associated with endothelial dysfunction in women. *Hypertension*, 1996. 28(4): p. 576-82.
[139] Jones, D.S., N.S. Andrawis, and D.R. Abernethy, Impaired endothelial-dependent forearm vascular relaxation in black Americans. *Clin Pharmacol Ther*, 1999. 65(4): p. 408-12.
[140] Gilligan, D.M., et al., Effects of estrogen replacement therapy on peripheral vasomotor function in postmenopausal women. *Am J Cardiol*, 1995. 75(4): p. 264-8.

[141] Herrington, D.M., et al., Endothelial-dependent coronary vasomotor responsiveness in postmenopausal women with and without estrogen replacement therapy. *Am J Cardiol,* 1994. 73(13): p. 951-2.
[142] Lieberman, E.H., et al., Estrogen improves endothelium-dependent, flow-mediated vasodilation in postmenopausal women. *Ann Intern Med*, 1994. 121(12): p. 936-41.
[143] Virdis, A., et al., Mechanisms responsible for endothelial dysfunction associated with acute estrogen deprivation in normotensive women. *Circulation*, 2000. 101(19): p. 2258-63.
[144] Taddei, S., et al., Endothelium-dependent forearm vasodilation is reduced in normotensive subjects with familial history of hypertension. *J Cardiovasc Pharmacol*, 1992. 20 Suppl 12: p. S193-5.
[145] Taddei, S., et al., Defective L-arginine-nitric oxide pathway in offspring of essential hypertensive patients. *Circulation*, 1996. 94(6): p. 1298-303.
[146] McAllister, A.S., et al., Basal nitric oxide production is impaired in offspring of patients with essential hypertension. *Clin Sci (Lond),* 1999. 97(2): p. 141-7.
[147] Panza, J.A., et al., Effect of antihypertensive treatment on endothelium-dependent vascular relaxation in patients with essential hypertension. *J Am Coll Cardiol,* 1993. 21(5): p. 1145-51.
[148] Millgard, J. and L. Lind, Acute hypertension impairs endothelium-dependent vasodilation. *Clin Sci (Lond),* 1998. 94(6): p. 601-7.
[149] Paniagua, O.A., M.B. Bryant, and J.A. Panza, Transient hypertension directly impairs endothelium-dependent vasodilation of the human microvasculature. *Hypertension*, 2000. 36(6): p. 941-4.
[150] Taddei, S., et al., Vasodilation to acetylcholine in primary and secondary forms of human hypertension. *Hypertension*, 1993. 21(6 Pt 2): p. 929-33.
[151] Schiffrin, E.L., et al., Antihypertensive effect of an endothelin receptor antagonist in DOCA-salt spontaneously hypertensive rats. *Br J Pharmacol*, 1995. 115(8): p. 1377-81.
[152] Schiffrin, E.L., et al., Correction of arterial structure and endothelial dysfunction in human essential hypertension by the angiotensin receptor antagonist losartan. *Circulation*, 2000. 101(14): p. 1653-9.
[153] Higashi, Y., et al., A comparison of angiotensin-converting enzyme inhibitors, calcium antagonists, beta-blockers and diuretic agents on reactive hyperemia in patients with essential hypertension: a multicenter study. *J Am Coll Cardiol,* 2000. 35(2): p. 284-91.
[154] Gao, Y.S., et al., Nebivolol induces endothelium-dependent relaxations of canine coronary arteries. *J Cardiovasc Pharmacol*, 1991. 17(6): p. 964-9.
[155] Cockcroft, J.R., et al., Nebivolol vasodilates human forearm vasculature: evidence for an L-arginine/NO-dependent mechanism. *J Pharmacol Exp Ther*, 1995. 274(3): p. 1067-71.
[156] Dawes, M., et al., The vasodilator action of nebivolol in forearm vasculature of subjects with essential hypertension. *Br J Clin Pharmacol*, 1999. 48(3): p. 460-3.
[157] Fargin, A., et al., The genomic clone G-21 which resembles a beta-adrenergic receptor sequence encodes the 5-HT1A receptor. *Nature*, 1988. 335(6188): p. 358-60.
[158] Kakoki, M., et al., Effects of vasodilatory beta-adrenoceptor antagonists on endothelium-derived nitric oxide release in rat kidney. *Hypertension*, 1999. 33(1 Pt 2): p. 467-71.

[159] Brehm, B.R., et al., Beta-blockers of the third generation inhibit endothelin-1 liberation, mRNA production and proliferation of human coronary smooth muscle and endothelial cells. *J Cardiovasc Pharmacol*, 2000. 36(5 Suppl 1): p. S401-3.

[160] Troost, R., et al., Nebivolol decreases systemic oxidative stress in healthy volunteers. Br J Clin Pharmacol, 2000. 50(4): p. 377-9.

[161] Tzemos, N., P.O. Lim, and T.M. MacDonald, Nebivolol reverses endothelial dysfunction in essential hypertension: a randomized, double-blind, crossover study. *Circulation*, 2001. 104(5): p. 511-4.

[162] Falskov, B., et al., Endothelial function is unaffected by changing between carvedilol and metoprolol in patients with heart failure--a randomized study. *Cardiovasc Diabetol*, 2011. 10: p. 91.

[163] Lindholm, L.H., et al., Cardiovascular morbidity and mortality in patients with diabetes in the Losartan Intervention For Endpoint reduction in hypertension study (LIFE): a randomised trial against atenolol. *Lancet*, 2002. 359(9311): p. 1004-10.

[164] Dahlof, B., et al., Cardiovascular morbidity and mortality in the Losartan Intervention For Endpoint reduction in hypertension study (LIFE): a randomised trial against atenolol. *Lancet*, 2002. 359(9311): p. 995-1003.

[165] Williams, B., et al., Differential impact of blood pressure-lowering drugs on central aortic pressure and clinical outcomes: principal results of the Conduit Artery Function Evaluation (CAFE) study. *Circulation*, 2006. 113(9): p. 1213-25.

[166] Kamp, O., G.T. Sieswerda, and C.A. Visser, Comparison of effects on systolic and diastolic left ventricular function of nebivolol versus atenolol in patients with uncomplicated essential hypertension. *Am J Cardiol*, 2003. 92(3): p. 344-8.

[167] Sorrentino, S.A., et al., Nebivolol exerts beneficial effects on endothelial function, early endothelial progenitor cells, myocardial neovascularization, and left ventricular dysfunction early after myocardial infarction beyond conventional beta1-blockade. *J Am Coll Cardiol*, 2011. 57(5): p. 601-11.

[168] Doerries, C., et al., Critical role of the NAD(P)H oxidase subunit p47phox for left ventricular remodeling/dysfunction and survival after myocardial infarction. *Circ Res*, 2007. 100(6): p. 894-903.

[169] Looi, Y.H., et al., Involvement of Nox2 NADPH oxidase in adverse cardiac remodeling after myocardial infarction. *Hypertension*, 2008. 51(2): p. 319-25.

[170] Brehm, B.R., et al., Effects of nebivolol on proliferation and apoptosis of human coronary artery smooth muscle and endothelial cells. *Cardiovasc Res,* 2001. 49(2): p. 430-9.

[171] Wolf, S.C., et al., Major differences in gene expression in human coronary smooth muscle cells after nebivolol or metoprolol treatment. *Int J Cardiol,* 2008. 125(1): p. 4-10.

[172] Taddei, S., et al., Forearm vasodilation in response to acetylcholine is increased by potassium in essential hypertensive patients. *J Hypertens Suppl,* 1993. 11(5): p. S144-5.

[173] Taddei, S., et al., Effect of potassium on vasodilation to acetylcholine in essential hypertension. *Hypertension*, 1994. 23(4): p. 485-90.

[174] Fang, J., S. Madhavan, and M.H. Alderman, Dietary potassium intake and stroke mortality. *Stroke*, 2000. 31(7): p. 1532-7.

[175] Farquharson, C.A. and A.D. Struthers, Spironolactone increases nitric oxide bioactivity, improves endothelial vasodilator dysfunction, and suppresses vascular angiotensin

I/angiotensin II conversion in patients with chronic heart failure. *Circulation*, 2000. 101(6): p. 594-7.
[176] Pitt, B., et al., The effect of spironolactone on morbidity and mortality in patients with severe heart failure. Randomized Aldactone Evaluation Study Investigators. *N Engl J Med,* 1999. 341(10): p. 709-17.
[177] Ullian, M.E., The role of corticosteriods in the regulation of vascular tone. *Cardiovasc Res*, 1999. 41(1): p. 55-64.
[178] Blanco-Rivero, J., et al., Participation of prostacyclin in endothelial dysfunction induced by aldosterone in normotensive and hypertensive rats. *Hypertension*, 2005. 46(1): p. 107-12.
[179] Garnier, A., et al., Cardiac specific increase in aldosterone production induces coronary dysfunction in aldosterone synthase-transgenic mice. *Circulation*, 2004. 110(13): p. 1819-25.
[180] Kobayashi, N., et al., Cardioprotective mechanisms of eplerenone on cardiac performance and remodeling in failing rat hearts. *Hypertension*, 2006. 47(4): p. 671-9.
[181] Nakamura, T., et al., Eplerenone potentiates protective effects of amlodipine against cardiovascular injury in salt-sensitive hypertensive rats. *Hypertens Res*, 2011. 34(7): p. 817-24.
[182] Fujimura, N., et al., Mineralocorticoid receptor blocker eplerenone improves endothelial function and inhibits Rho-associated kinase activity in patients with hypertension. *Clin Pharmacol Ther*, 2012. 91(2): p. 289-97.
[183] Savoia, C., et al., Selective mineralocorticoid receptor blocker eplerenone reduces resistance artery stiffness in hypertensive patients. *Hypertension*, 2008. 51(2): p. 432-9.
[184] Imanishi, T., et al., Addition of eplerenone to an angiotensin-converting enzyme inhibitor effectively improves nitric oxide bioavailability. *Hypertension*, 2008. 51(3): p. 734-41.
[185] McMurray, J.J., et al., ESC Guidelines for the diagnosis and treatment of acute and chronic heart failure 2012: The Task Force for the Diagnosis and Treatment of Acute and Chronic Heart Failure 2012 of the European Society of Cardiology. Developed in collaboration with the Heart Failure Association (HFA) of the ESC. *Eur Heart J*, 2012. 33(14): p. 1787-847.
[186] Hansson, L., et al., Randomised trial of effects of calcium antagonists compared with diuretics and beta-blockers on cardiovascular morbidity and mortality in hypertension: the Nordic Diltiazem (NORDIL) study. *Lancet*, 2000. 356(9227): p. 359-65.
[187] Brown, M.J., et al., Morbidity and mortality in patients randomised to double-blind treatment with a long-acting calcium-channel blocker or diuretic in the International Nifedipine GITS study: Intervention as a Goal in Hypertension Treatment (INSIGHT). *Lancet*, 2000. 356(9227): p. 366-72.
[188] Lyons, D., J. Webster, and N. Benjamin, The effect of antihypertensive therapy on responsiveness to local intra-arterial NG-monomethyl-L-arginine in patients with essential hypertension. *J Hypertens,* 1994. 12(9): p. 1047-52.
[189] Perticone, F., et al., Calcium antagonist isradipine improves abnormal endothelium-dependent vasodilation in never treated hypertensive patients. *Cardiovasc Res*, 1999. 41(1): p. 299-306.
[190] Taddei, S., et al., Lacidipine restores endothelium-dependent vasodilation in essential hypertensive patients. *Hypertension*, 1997. 30(6): p. 1606-12.

[191] Yamamoto, E., et al., Calcium channel blockers, more than diuretics, enhance vascular protective effects of angiotensin receptor blockers in salt-loaded hypertensive rats. *PLoS One*, 2012. 7(6): p. e39162.

[192] Schiffrin, E.L. and L.Y. Deng, Structure and function of resistance arteries of hypertensive patients treated with a beta-blocker or a calcium channel antagonist. *J Hypertens*, 1996. 14(10): p. 1247-55.

[193] Frielingsdorf, J., et al., Normalization of abnormal coronary vasomotion by calcium antagonists in patients with hypertension. *Circulation*, 1996. 93(7): p. 1380-7.

[194] Effect of nifedipine and cerivastatin on coronary endothelial function in patients with coronary artery disease: the ENCORE I Study (Evaluation of Nifedipine and Cerivastatin On Recovery of coronary Endothelial function). *Circulation*, 2003. 107(3): p. 422-8.

[195] Luscher, T.F., et al., A randomized placebo-controlled study on the effect of nifedipine on coronary endothelial function and plaque formation in patients with coronary artery disease: the ENCORE II study. *Eur Heart J,* 2009. 30(13): p. 1590-7.

[196] Rubanyi, G.M. and P.M. Vanhoutte, Calcium and activation of the release of endothelium-derived relaxing factor. *Ann N Y Acad Sci,* 1988. 522: p. 226-33.

[197] Lupo, E., et al., In vitro antioxidant activity of calcium antagonists against LDL oxidation compared with alpha-tocopherol. *Biochem Biophys Res Commun*, 1994. 203(3): p. 1803-8.

[198] van Amsterdam, F.T., et al., Lacidipine: a dihydropyridine calcium antagonist with antioxidant activity. *Free Radic Biol Med,* 1992. 12(3): p. 183-7.

[199] Haynes, W.G., et al., Pharmacology of endothelin-1 in vivo in humans. *J Cardiovasc Pharmacol*, 1991. 17 Suppl 7: p. S284-6.

[200] Kiowski, W., et al., Endothelin-1-induced vasoconstriction in humans. Reversal by calcium channel blockade but not by nitrovasodilators or endothelium-derived relaxing factor. *Circulation*, 1991. 83(2): p. 469-75.

[201] Kiowski, W. and L. Linder, Reversal of endothelin-1-induced vasoconstriction by nifedipine in human resistance vessels in vivo in healthy subjects. *Am J Cardiol*, 1992. 69(12): p. 1063-6.

[202] Cardillo, C., et al., Role of endothelin in the increased vascular tone of patients with essential hypertension. *Hypertension*, 1999. 33(2): p. 753-8.

[203] Raij, L., Hypertension, endothelium, and cardiovascular risk factors. *Am J Med*, 1991. 90(2A): p. 13S-18S.

[204] Tiryaki, O., et al., Effects of lisinopril, irbesartan, and amlodipine on the thrombogenic variables in the early and late stages of the treatment in hypertensive patients. *Clin Exp Hypertens*, 2012. 34(2): p. 145-52.

[205] Goldblatt, H., et al., Studies on Experimental Hypertension : I. The Production of Persistent Elevation of Systolic Blood Pressure by Means of Renal Ischemia. *J Exp Med*, 1934. 59(3): p. 347-79.

[206] Dzau, V.J., Local expression and pathophysiological role of renin-angiotensin in the blood vessels and heart. *Basic Res Cardiol*, 1993. 88 Suppl 1: p. 1-14.

[207] Siragy, H.M., M. de Gasparo, and R.M. Carey, Angiotensin type 2 receptor mediates valsartan-induced hypotension in conscious rats. *Hypertension*, 2000. 35(5): p. 1074-7.

[208] Erdos, E.G., The angiotensin I converting enzyme. *Fed Proc*, 1977. 36(5): p. 1760-5.

[209] Zhang, X., et al., Role of endothelial kinins in control of coronary nitric oxide production. Hypertension, 1997. 30(5): p. 1105-11.
[210] Vanhoutte, P.M., [Endothelial dysfunction and coronary heart disease. Interaction of endothelium and thrombocytes]. *Schweiz Rundsch Med Prax,* 1993. 82(42): p. 1161-6.
[211] Hornig, B., C. Kohler, and H. Drexler, Role of bradykinin in mediating vascular effects of angiotensin-converting enzyme inhibitors in humans. *Circulation*, 1997. 95(5): p. 1115-8.
[212] Anderson, T.J., et al., Comparative study of ACE-inhibition, angiotensin II antagonism, and calcium channel blockade on flow-mediated vasodilation in patients with coronary disease (BANFF study). *J Am Coll Cardiol*, 2000. 35(1): p. 60-6.
[213] Mancini, G.B., et al., Angiotensin-converting enzyme inhibition with quinapril improves endothelial vasomotor dysfunction in patients with coronary artery disease. The TREND (Trial on Reversing ENdothelial Dysfunction) Study. *Circulation*, 1996. 94(3): p. 258-65.
[214] Schiffrin, E.L., Remodeling of resistance arteries in human hypertension: effects of cilazapril, an angiotensin-I-converting enzyme inhibitor. *Cardiology*, 1995. 86 Suppl 1: p. 16-22.
[215] Rizzoni, D., et al., Effects of long-term antihypertensive treatment with lisinopril on resistance arteries in hypertensive patients with left ventricular hypertrophy. *J Hypertens,* 1997. 15(2): p. 197-204.
[216] Antony, I., G. Lerebours, and A. Nitenberg, Angiotensin-converting enzyme inhibition restores flow-dependent and cold pressor test-induced dilations in coronary arteries of hypertensive patients. *Circulation*, 1996. 94(12): p. 3115-22.
[217] Taddei, S., et al., Effects of angiotensin converting enzyme inhibition on endothelium-dependent vasodilatation in essential hypertensive patients. *J Hypertens*, 1998. 16(4): p. 447-56.
[218] Kiowski, W., et al., Effects of cilazapril on vascular structure and function in essential hypertension. *Hypertension*, 1996. 27(3 Pt 1): p. 371-6.
[219] Creager, M.A. and M.A. Roddy, Effect of captopril and enalapril on endothelial function in hypertensive patients. *Hypertension*, 1994. 24(4): p. 499-505.
[220] Hirooka, Y., et al., Captopril improves impaired endothelium-dependent vasodilation in hypertensive patients. *Hypertension*, 1992. 20(2): p. 175-80.
[221] Millgard, J., et al., Captopril, but not nifedipine, improves endothelium-dependent vasodilation in hypertensive patients. *J Hum Hypertens*, 1998. 12(8): p. 511-6.
[222] Prasad, A., et al., Acute and chronic angiotensin-1 receptor antagonism reverses endothelial dysfunction in atherosclerosis. *Circulation*, 2000. 101(20): p. 2349-54.
[223] Ghiadoni, L., et al., Effect of the angiotensin II type 1 receptor blocker candesartan on endothelial function in patients with essential hypertension. *Hypertension*, 2000. 35(1 Pt 2): p. 501-6.
[224] Tzemos, N., P.O. Lim, and T.M. MacDonald, Valsartan improves endothelial dysfunction in hypertension: a randomized, double-blind study. *Cardiovasc Ther*, 2009. 27(3): p. 151-8.
[225] Hirooka, Y., et al., Effects of valsartan or amlodipine on endothelial function and oxidative stress after one year follow-up in patients with essential hypertension. *Clin Exp Hypertens*, 2008. 30(3): p. 267-76.

[226] Kerth, P.A. and P.M. Vanhoutte, Effects of perindoprilat on endothelium-dependent relaxations and contractions in isolated blood vessels. *Am J Hypertens,* 1991. 4(3 Pt 2): p. 226S-234S.

[227] Ceconi, C., et al., ACE inhibition with perindopril and endothelial function. Results of a substudy of the EUROPA study: PERTINENT. *Cardiovasc Res*, 2007. 73(1): p. 237-46.

[228] Miyamoto, M., et al., The effect of antihypertensive drugs on endothelial function as assessed by flow-mediated vasodilation in hypertensive patients. *Int J Vasc Med,* 2012. 2012: p. 453264.

[229] Terashima, M., et al., Protective effect of telmisartan against endothelial dysfunction after coronary drug-eluting stent implantation in hypertensive patients. *JACC Cardiovasc Interv,* 2012. 5(2): p. 182-90.

[230] Chou, C.L., et al., Direct renin inhibitor prevents and ameliorates insulin resistance, aortic endothelial dysfunction and vascular remodeling in fructose-fed hypertensive rats. *Hypertens Res*, 2012.

[231] Virdis, A., et al., Effect of aliskiren treatment on endothelium-dependent vasodilation and aortic stiffness in essential hypertensive patients. *Eur Heart J*, 2012. 33(12): p. 1530-8.

[232] Cherney, D.Z., et al., The Effect of Direct Renin Inhibition Alone and in Combination With ACE Inhibition on Endothelial Function, Arterial Stiffness, and Renal Function in Type 1 Diabetes. *Diabetes* Care, 2012.

[233] Yanagisawa, M., et al., A novel peptide vasoconstrictor, endothelin, is produced by vascular endothelium and modulates smooth muscle Ca2+ channels. *J Hypertens Suppl*, 1988. 6(4): p. S188-91.

[234] Haynes, W.G., F.E. Strachan, and D.J. Webb, Endothelin ETA and ETB receptors cause vasoconstriction of human resistance and capacitance vessels in vivo. *Circulation*, 1995. 92(3): p. 357-63.

[235] Imai, T., et al., Induction of endothelin-1 gene by angiotensin and vasopressin in endothelial cells. *Hypertension*, 1992. 19(6 Pt 2): p. 753-7.

[236] d'Uscio, L.V., et al., Structure and function of small arteries in salt-induced hypertension: effects of chronic endothelin-subtype-A-receptor blockade. *Hypertension*, 1997. 30(4): p. 905-11.

[237] Kohno, M., et al., Plasma immunoreactive endothelin in essential hypertension. *Am J Med*, 1990. 88(6): p. 614-8.

[238] Russell, F.D., J.N. Skepper, and A.P. Davenport, Endothelin peptide and converting enzymes in human endothelium. *J Cardiovasc Pharmacol*, 1998. 31 Suppl 1: p. S19-21.

[239] Wagner, O.F., et al., Polar secretion of endothelin-1 by cultured endothelial cells. *J Biol Chem*, 1992. 267(23): p. 16066-8.

[240] Schiffrin, E.L., et al., Enhanced expression of endothelin-1 gene in resistance arteries in severe human essential hypertension. *J Hypertens*, 1997. 15(1): p. 57-63.

[241] Ergul, S., et al., Racial differences in plasma endothelin-1 concentrations in individuals with essential hypertension. *Hypertension*, 1996. 28(4): p. 652-5.

[242] Krum, H., et al., The effect of an endothelin-receptor antagonist, bosentan, on blood pressure in patients with essential hypertension. Bosentan Hypertension Investigators. *N Engl J Med*, 1998. 338(12): p. 784-90.

[243] Reriani, M., et al., Long-term administration of endothelin receptor antagonist improves coronary endothelial function in patients with early atherosclerosis. *Circulation*, 2010. 122(10): p. 958-66.
[244] Liang, F., et al., Ambrisentan and tadalafil synergistically relax endothelin-induced contraction of rat pulmonary arteries. *Hypertension*, 2012. 59(3): p. 705-11.
[245] Halls, M.L., R.A. Bathgate, and R.J. Summers, Comparison of signaling pathways activated by the relaxin family peptide receptors, RXFP1 and RXFP2, using reporter genes. *J Pharmacol Exp Ther,* 2007. 320(1): p. 281-90.
[246] Dschietzig, T., et al., Relaxin, a pregnancy hormone, is a functional endothelin-1 antagonist: attenuation of endothelin-1-mediated vasoconstriction by stimulation of endothelin type-B receptor expression via ERK-1/2 and nuclear factor-kappaB. Circ Res, 2003. 92(1): p. 32-40.
[247] Burnett, J.C., Jr., Vasopeptidase inhibition: a new concept in blood pressure management. J Hypertens Suppl, 1999. 17(1): p. S37-43.
[248] Erdos, E.G. and R.A. Skidgel, Neutral endopeptidase 24.11 (enkephalinase) and related regulators of peptide hormones. *FASEB J*, 1989. 3(2): p. 145-51.
[249] Burnett, J.C., Jr., et al., Atrial natriuretic peptide elevation in congestive heart failure in the human. *Science*, 1986. 231(4742): p. 1145-7.
[250] Wei, C.M., et al., Atrial natriuretic peptide and C-type natriuretic peptide in spontaneously hypertensive rats and their vasorelaxing actions in vitro. *Hypertension*, 1994. 23(6 Pt 2): p. 903-7.
[251] Tikkanen, T., et al., Dual inhibition of neutral endopeptidase and angiotensin-converting enzyme in rats with hypertension and diabetes mellitus. *Hypertension*, 1998. 32(4): p. 778-85.
[252] d'Uscio, L.V., et al., Vasopeptidase Inhibition Prevents Endothelial Dysfunction of Resistance Arteries in Salt-Sensitive Hypertension in Comparison With Single ACE Inhibition. *Hypertension*, 2001. 37(1): p. 28-33.
[253] Trippodo, N.C., et al., Effects of omapatrilat in low, normal, and high renin experimental hypertension. *Am J Hypertens*, 1998. 11(3 Pt 1): p. 363-72.
[254] Quaschning, T., et al., Vasopeptidase inhibition restores renovascular endothelial dysfunction in salt-induced hypertension. *J Am Soc Nephrol*, 2001. 12(11): p. 2280-7.
[255] Maniu, C.V., D.M. Meyer, and M.M. Redfield, Hemodynamic and humoral effects of vasopeptidase inhibition in canine hypertension. *Hypertension*, 2002. 40(4): p. 528-34.
[256] Cheng, Z.J., et al., Vascular and renal effects of vasopeptidase inhibition and angiotensin-converting enzyme blockade in spontaneously diabetic Goto-Kakizaki rats. *J Hypertens,* 2005. 23(9): p. 1757-70.
[257] Taddei, S., et al., Vitamin C improves endothelium-dependent vasodilation by restoring nitric oxide activity in essential hypertension. *Circulation*, 1998. 97(22): p. 2222-9.
[258] Frei, B., L. England, and B.N. Ames, Ascorbate is an outstanding antioxidant in human blood plasma. *Proc Natl Acad Sci U S A,* 1989. 86(16): p. 6377-81.
[259] Solzbach, U., et al., Vitamin C improves endothelial dysfunction of epicardial coronary arteries in hypertensive patients. *Circulation*, 1997. 96(5): p. 1513-9.
[260] Jeserich, M., et al., Vitamin C improves endothelial function of epicardial coronary arteries in patients with hypercholesterolaemia or essential hypertension--assessed by cold pressor testing. *Eur Heart J*, 1999. 20(22): p. 1676-80.

[261] Engler, M.M., et al., Antioxidant vitamins C and E improve endothelial function in children with hyperlipidemia: Endothelial Assessment of Risk from Lipids in Youth (EARLY) Trial. *Circulation*, 2003. 108(9): p. 1059-63.

[262] Lovat, L.B., et al., Double-blind trial of vitamin C in elderly hypertensives. *J Hum Hypertens*, 1993. 7(4): p. 403-5.

[263] Ghosh, S.K., et al., A double-blind, placebo-controlled parallel trial of vitamin C treatment in elderly patients with hypertension. *Gerontology*, 1994. 40(5): p. 268-72.

[264] Duffy, S.J., et al., Treatment of hypertension with ascorbic acid. *Lancet*, 1999. 354(9195): p. 2048-9.

[265] Fotherby, M.D., et al., Effect of vitamin C on ambulatory blood pressure and plasma lipids in older persons. *J Hypertens*, 2000. 18(4): p. 411-5.

[266] Wray, D.W., et al., Acute reversal of endothelial dysfunction in the elderly after antioxidant consumption. *Hypertension*, 2012. 59(4): p. 818-24.

[267] Garcia, C.E., et al., Effect of copper-zinc superoxide dismutase on endothelium-dependent vasodilation in patients with essential hypertension. *Hypertension*, 1995. 26(6 Pt 1): p. 863-8.

[268] Nakazono, K., et al., Does superoxide underlie the pathogenesis of hypertension? Proc Natl Acad Sci U S A, 1991. 88(22): p. 10045-8.

[269] Cardillo, C., et al., Xanthine oxidase inhibition with oxypurinol improves endothelial vasodilator function in hypercholesterolemic but not in hypertensive patients. *Hypertension*, 1997. 30(1 Pt 1): p. 57-63.

[270] Kris-Etherton, P.M., et al., Antioxidant vitamin supplements and cardiovascular disease. *Circulation*, 2004. 110(5): p. 637-41.

[271] Traupe, T., et al., Distinct roles of estrogen receptors alpha and beta mediating acute vasodilation of epicardial coronary arteries. *Hypertension*, 2007. 49(6): p. 1364-70.

[272] Meyer, M.R., et al., Deletion of G protein-coupled estrogen receptor increases endothelial vasoconstriction. *Hypertension*, 2012. 59(2): p. 507-12.

[273] Zhou, S., et al., Repression of P66Shc expression by SIRT1 contributes to the prevention of hyperglycemia-induced endothelial dysfunction. *Circ Res*, 2011. 109(6): p. 639-48.

[274] Mitsutake, Y., et al., Coronary endothelial dysfunction distal to stent of first-generation drug-eluting stents. *JACC Cardiovasc Interv,* 2012. 5(9): p. 966-73.

[275] Plass, C.A., et al., Time course of endothelium-dependent and -independent coronary vasomotor response to coronary balloons and stents. Comparison of plain and drug-eluting balloons and stents. *JACC Cardiovasc Interv*, 2012. 5(7): p. 741-51.

[276] Matsue, Y., et al., Endothelial dysfunction measured by peripheral arterial tonometry predicts prognosis in patients with heart failure with preserved ejection fraction. *Int J Cardiol*, 2012.

In: Arterial Hypertension
Editors: Marten Vosler and Siemen Weber
ISBN: 978-1-62417-852-8
© 2013 Nova Science Publishers, Inc.

Chapter 2

Masked Arterial Hypertension: Less Known, but Important

Goran Koracevic
Department for Cardiovascular Diseases, Clinical Center Nis,
Medical Faculty, University of Nis, Serbia

Abstract

In the early 2000s, masked hypertension (MAHT) was originally defined by Thomas Pickering as the hypertensive condition undetectable by conventional blood pressure (BP) measurements in the clinic or office environment. Thus, MAHT is an elevated ambulatory or home BP in the absence of increased office BP.

The best way to diagnose MAHT is to use ambulatory BP monitoring (ABPM), because sleep-time BP can not be measured otherwise noninvasively. MAHT is an emerging clinical entity predisposing to subclinical organ damage and to increased cardiovascular risk.

MAHT prevalence has been estimated to be 10-38%. MAHT is prevalent and may be even more so: as home BP measurement becomes more popular, the detection MAHT will increase. MAHT is more frequently found in pre-hypertensive individuals. Recent study showed a MAHT prevalence of 8.1%; and older age, high-normal systolic and diastolic office BP, greater BMI, current smoking, diabetes, and electrocardiographic LVH were found to be independently correlated to MAHT.

According to some authors, there are basically two types of MAHT: 1) MAHT in general population (10-15%, which makes hundred millions in the world) -in people with normal office BP, but elevated out-of-office BP (e.g. at workplace). 2) The other type of MAHT occurs in about 30% of patients with sustained („classic") AHT, who have diagnosed AHT and apparently well-controlled BP (by therapy), i.e. normal office BP, but not normal BP all day long, e.g. BP is not controlled in the morning and/or in the night). Other authors believe that only the first type is MAHT, while the second is only "insufficiently efficient antihypertensive therapy."

Classification of MAHT into subtypes, according to BP circadian cycle (morning hypertension, daytime hypertension, and night-time hypertension regardless of the presence of antihypertensive treatment) has been recently proposed. MAHT carries nearly the same cardiovascular risks as sustained hypertension. In 2012 study, multivariate regression analyses revealed that the presence of MAHT was one of the independent determinants of LVH, carotid atherosclerosis, and albuminuria.

According to currently available medical literature, MAHT is prevalent, prognostically important, associated with subclinical damages and treatable form of hypertension, but insufficiently recognized entity.

1. Introduction

As early as 70 years ago it was described that *office blood pressure (BP) can vary by as much as 25 mmHg between visits* [1]. The precise measurement of BP continues to be the most important technique for the assessment of the arterial hypertension (AHT) and its outcomes, and proofs are accumulating that the traditional office BP measurement technique may yield inadequate or misleading estimates of a subject's true BP status [1]. Conventional procedure for BP measurement is *grossly misleading* [2]. Clinic (office) BP provides an incomplete and potentially ambiguous assessment of the severity of AHT also in African Americans with hypertensive kidney disease, largely due to the increased nighttime BP [3].

The limitations of office BP estimation result from at least 4 sources:

1) *the inherent variability of BP*, together with the *small number of readings* which are typically taken in the doctor's office,
2) *poor technique* (e.g., terminal digit preference, rapid cuff deflation, inadequate cuff and bladder size),
3) *the white coat effect* (the increase of BP that occurs in the medical care environment), and
4) *the masked effect* (a decrease of BP in treated hypertensives, that happens in doctor's office), which may lead to under-treatment; in the another population – without antihypertensives, but with „masked" hypertension (MAHT), the resting, office BP is normal, but out-of-office, ambulatory BP is elevated or substantially lower [1].

Furthermore, *O'Brien* reviews the following shortcomings of office BP measurement. Firstly, office BP measurement itself (being stressogenic) creates the phenomenon of *white coat hypertension (WC-AHT), which affects as many as 20% of patients with AHT*, diagnosed by conventional measurement. Secondly, (resting) *office BP assessment fails to detect AHT in ≈10–20% of the general population (MAHT),* which if *even conservatively estimated at 5% translates into as many as 10 million people in the USA* [2]. Thus, the diagnosis of AHT *with conventional office BP measurement may be incorrect in as many as a 1/3 of all subjects.* One of the shortcomings of the conventional office measurement for defining BP status is that it is not informative about nocturnal AHT, which is one of the most sensitive predictors of cardiovascular (CV) events. Additionally, *treatment of AHT should cover 24 hours and it is largely wasted unless BP is controlled.* Treated patients with uncontrolled BP have a CV risk only modestly less than that of untreated individuals [2]. Importantly, elevations of BP in the clinical environment, at home, and while ambulatory seem to have an additive effect on CV risk [4].

Improvements in BP assessment take two forms at the present time: by *improving the office BP technique* (e.g., using accurate validated automated monitors that can easily perform multiple readings), and by *using out-of-office monitoring* to supplement the BP values taken in the doctor's office. Out-of-office monitoring can be twofold: *self (or home) (HBPM) and ambulatory BP monitoring (ABPM).* While *both modalities have been available for 30 years*, only now are they recognized as important and finding their way into routine clinical practice [1].

The addition of ABPM to traditional office BP assessment has complicated the process, because the separation of normotension and AHT can be assessed independently by each of the 2 methods. We thus have 4 potential groups of subjects who are, first, normotensive by both methods (*true normotensives*); second, hypertensive by both (true, or *sustained, hypertensives*); third, hypertensive by office assessment and normotensive by ambulatory measurement (*white-coat hypertensives*); and, fourth, normotensive by office assessment and hypertensive by ambulatory measurement (*MAHT*). From a clinical point of view, the first 2 groups are easy to deal with, because both methods give the same result of classification. Of more interest are the groups in which there is disagreement. The third group (usually referred to as WC-AHT) has been extensively studied and is generally accepted as being at relatively low risk of CV morbidity. This view is consistent with the *concept that ambulatory BP* (being far longer, among other advantages) *is a better predictor of risk than office BP* [5]. Until now, little attention has been given to the fourth group, whose condition has been given the titles of "*reverse WC-AHT* " or "*white-coat normotension.*" *If it is true that the ambulatory BP gives the better classification of risk, it would imply that these people should be regarded as being genuinely hypertensive (because their prognosis is closer to hypertensives than to normotensives)* [5].

Improvements in AHT diagnostics are very important, having in mind extremely high prevalence of the disease worldwide. Moreover, AHT prevalence is expected to raise. It is projected that the proportion of the older population (aged ≥65 years) in Europe will increase from 20% in 2000 to 35% in 2050. The prevalence of AHT increases with aging to the point where >1/2 of people aged 60-69 years and ≈3/4 of those aged ≥70 years have AHT [2].

The physician should recognize that it is much easier to suspect the diagnosis of WC-AHT, as individuals will usually declare normal BP at home. In contrast, MAHT needs to be looked for and there are very few clinical hints as to its presence. Prevalence of MAHT and WC-AHT seems to be similar – this is a fact which clearly documents that *MAHT is often overlooked* [6]. A normal office BP does not mean that a subject is not at risk from an elevated BP, which can occur at other times of the day (when one does not measure it). On the other hand, whether MAHT is a definite clinical trait is still a matter of debate, because only 71% of individuals with MAHT according to the first ABPM session confirmed this pattern in the second ABPM. No studies reviewed in the present analysis defined the MAHT phenotype by repeated ABPM [7].

2. Definition

MAHT is an increased ambulatory or home BP in the absence of elevated BP in the clinical setting, i.e. with a normal office BP of <140/90 mmHg [5, 8]. MAHT (*isolated ambulatory AHT*), was *first described by Devereux and Pickering* in *1991* as "*white-coat normotension*" (because it is the *opposite of WC-AHT)* [9, 10]. *Pickering* et al. also proposed the term "masked hypertension" [5, 6]. The same entity has been described occasionally as: "*reversed WC-AHT* " [6, 11], or *"isolated office BP control"* [12] or *"occult workplace AHT"* [5, 13].

More precisely, *MAHT is defined by elevated daytime (≥135/85 mmHg) or increased nighttime (≥120/70 mmHg) AMBP in those with controlled office BP (<140/90 mmHg)* [3]. MAHT also can be defined as a *daytime ambulatory dBP >85 mmHg and a clinic BP <85 mmHg* [5]. MAHT is an emerging clinical entity, which predispose to subclinical organ damage and to increased CV risk [7].

Patients with WC-AHT had normal ambulatory BP monitoring values, although these were somewhat higher than in the normotensive group. Similarly, both CV mortality and morbidity were somewhat elevated (numerically) in subjects with WC-AHT, but these levels did not reach statistical significance. In contrast, patients with *MAHT had a risk that was double that of normotensive subjects* and close to patients with sustained AHT. These results were independent of gender, use of antihypertensive medication, and risk-factor score. Paradoxically, *although more dangerous, MAHT is a much less well-known* entity, which seems to carry a distinctly more serious prognosis [6].

Unlike most forms of essential AHT, clinic readings in MAHT in the morning are commonly lower than those obtained during the rest of the day (14). *MAHT definition should be limited to untreated individuals* with office BP values <140/90mmHg and elevated self-measured BP (i.e. home BP>135/85mmHg) or ambulatory BP (i.e. average 24-hour BP >125/80 mmHg, or daytime BP >135/85 mmHg). In *treated* AHT patients, normal office BP values in the presence of elevated outside office BP *should not identify MAHT, but rather* a condition of *incomplete BP control* during daily activities or at night (which is undetected by conventional BP measurements, performed by the physician) [7, 15].

Moreover, the usage of 24-hour ABPM in prehypertensive subjects found that *prehypertension is not a homogeneous BP type*. More specifically, this is a *mixed condition,* composed by 2 groups of *prehypertensive subjects: with normal ABPM values (actual prehypertensives)* and *with increased ABPM recordings (MAHT)* [16, 17].

Numerous studies revealed that *prehypertension* is linked to the target-organ damage (TOD). For example, prehypertensive subjects had higher left ventricular (LV) mass then normotensives. Furthermore, the Strong Heart Study discovered that prehypertensive participants had higher LV mass, LV wall thickness and relative LV wall thickness than their normotensive counterparts. Additionally, some results suggested that arterial functions were impaired at the prehypertensive BP range. Moreover, prehypertension is associated with thickening of the intimal layer of radial artery [17].

Prehypertensives with MAHT have higher common carotid artery-intimal medial thickness (*CCA-IMT*) values than actual prehypertensives and normotensives. Furthermore, the lack of statistical difference between actual prehypertensives and normotensives regarding CCA-IMT, leads to the hypothesis that the reported links of prehypertension with CCA-IMT may be attributed to the *high prevalence of MAHT (24.8%) among prehypertensive individuals.* This finding imposes a need *of ABPM monitoring use in prehypertensive patients*, for the early identification of MAHT and a better prognostication [17].

MAHT is defined as good in-office BP control <140/90 mmHg, but with daytime ABPM or home sBP ≥135 mmHg or dBP ≥85 mmHg. Some authorities incorporate *nocturnal* BPs into the definition of MAHT and argue that an *averaged sleep sBP value of >120 mmHg also constitutes MAHT when office BP is controlled* [18].

3. Causes and Interpretation of MAHT

Generally, there are 2 groups of factors to explain MAHT, which are not mutually exclusive:

1. The *resting* office BP could be relatively low as compared to the ambulatory BP, when the *physician's presence creates an atmosphere of security and trust,* in contrast to BP that affect the individual's situation at work or at home, with the result that BP measurements are lower in the doctor's office; or
2. There could be factors that selectively raise the ambulatory BP. For example, *smokers* tend to have high daytime ambulatory BP (when they are likely to be smoking) in comparison with their office BP (when they do not smoke). Also, subjects who are *more physically active* during the day will tend to have higher daytime BP [5].

Moreover, a recent study of 1459 untreated Finnish adult individuals revealed a MAHT prevalence of 8.1%. *Older age, high-normal office sBP and dBP, greater body mass index (BMI), current smoking and diabetes mellitus (DM)* were independently correlated to MAHT presence [7, 19]. MAHT is prevalent in patients with *chronic kidney disease (CKD), DM,* and *obstructive sleep apnea (OSA)* [20]. Conditions related to MAHT include: *smoking, DM, CKD, microalbuminuria,* LV hypertrophy *(LVH)* and *OSA* [3, 20-23]. LVH and microalbuminuria are merely the consequence of MAHT than a cause.

MAHT in youth is associated with *obesity* and *increased LVMI* [24]. MAHT is more frequent in *men* of increasing age [25, 26]. Aging increases both ambulatory and clinic BP, *but the rate of increase of office BP is greater than that of ambulatory BP* [24]. Therefore, *office BP is more likely to exceed ambulatory BP in elderly individuals* [8, 27]. Consequently, elderly individuals are candidates for WC-AHT. The higher MAHT prevalence in *older males* was confirmed in a recent study of 2370 workers. Participants had BP measured in the workplace and by ABPM. The prevalence was higher in *men* (adjusted odds ratio [OR], 2.38), and in men the prevalence increased with *age* (OR, 2.08 for 40–49 years; adjusted OR, 1.91 for ≥50 years of age), a *BMI ≥27* (adjusted OR, 1.78) and when *alcohol* intake exceeded 6 drinks per week (OR, 2.12) [26].

Patients with MAHT tended to be *male, past smokers* and *older*, and they had consumed more *alcohol* [5]. Numerous factors selectively affecting ambulatory BP include *young* age, *male* gender, and *smoking* [12]. Several factors have been reported to contribute to MAHT (e.g., *smoking, alcohol drinking, physical activity*, and *stress*) [28]. In addition, it has been recognized that the prevalence of MAHT is high in outpatients with *DM* [8, 22, 29, 30]. Risk factors for MAHT are: the use of *alcohol, tobacco,* and *caffeine* as well as *physical inactivity* [6]. In a study of Charvat et al., *BMI* was significantly higher in patients with MAHT. *The significantly higher BP elevation during exercise in overweight subjects could be one of the explanations for MAHT during the daily hours* [31].

Type 2 DM patients had higher CCA-IMT if they had MAHT, detected by ABPM, as compared to those with normal BP during daily hours. Increased arterial stiffness is linked to MAHT, too, which could be supported by significantly higher pulse pressure during 24-hour ABPM [31].

It is important for practice to know about the "*masking effect*" in AHT (i.e., controlled office BP, but uncontrolled ambulatory BP *despite antihypertensive therapy*). One of the reasons for such „masking effect" is that antihypertensive drug do not encompass a full 24-hour period. Because an individual patient takes the medication in the morning, a couple of hours later, in the physician's office, BP values are usually normal, but they may be substantially elevated during stress or physical effort, or at the end of the dosing interval (i.e., during the night and early morning hours) [6].

Thus, in many hypertensive patients, office BP is seemingly well controlled, but early morning BP (which is very important), before the patients take the medication, may be uncontrolled, thereby accelerating the CV risk. *DM, CKD* and *stroke* are risk factors for high morning home BP. Therefore, more intensive treatment is needed to achieve the therapeutic goal in such patients [32]. On the other hand, taking antihypertensive drugs solely in the morning (versus taking them twice a day) was associated with a higher probability of office resistance and underestimation of BP control. This may be partially because of the fact that most BP determinations occurred in the morning [12]. MAHT (more precisely: „masking effect") commonly occur in *treated* AHT patients, but is not persistent phenomenon and probably results from an *accidentally low office BP value on one particular occasion* [33]. Notably, the ratio of MAHT in AHT patients with DM was significantly higher than that in AHT patients without DM. Thus, more aggressive BP treatment, particularly for the reduction of morning home sBP, would be needed in AHT patients with DM. Indeed, the clinical significance of morning home BP in patients with type 2 DM has been well recognized [32, 34-36].

Several population studies have compared office and ambulatory BP. Depending on the subjects studied, some have shown daytime BP to be a little higher than clinic BP, whereas others have found the reverse. One important finding from an Italian population study has been that the *ambulatory BP shows much less increase with age than the clinic BP*. In a Danish study, 86% of men 42 years of age had daytime BP higher than the clinic BP, whereas this was true of only 51% at the age of 72 years. The *white-coat effect* (higher office than ambulatory BP) is hence more marked in *older* people, and because *MAHT is equivalent to a negative white-coat effect*, it is reasonable to suppose that AHT *would be less prevalent with increasing age* [5].

Occupational strain or stress is a result of a combination of high demands with low decision latitude in the workplace, and there is accumulating evidence, which links it with BP elevation and CV diseases. The demands of the workplace incorporate both job- and human-related variables. Job-related variables include work schedules (shift work or irregular hours, rotating schedules), time pressures, machine-paced work, repetitive-routine or monotonous activities; physical conditions such as heat, noise, lighting, sedentary or active tasks; contact with the public; solitary or interactive tasks, hierarchical status (involving different degrees of responsibility, decision authority and autonomy, and prestige), etc. Stress may also stem from problematic relationships with co-workers or superiors, such as conflicts or unfair treatment, ambiguous or contradictory work demands, and role overload or under-stimulation. To the contrary, support from colleagues or supervisors may alleviate stress. Human variables that impact on stress are job satisfaction, the organization of the work, and whether the job offers security and flexibility, recognition and reward, and possibilities for advancement. Personal variables, such as self-perceived capabilities, self-confidence, and the ability to cope with stressful situations, are important, too. Indeed, it has been suggested that the perception that one's job is stressful or the perception of control over events may be powerful predictors of elevated BP [37].

MAHT is a common feature in type 2 DM patients being treated for AHT. The observed relation with sodium intake raised the hypothesis that *excessive sodium intake* may play a part in the genesis of MAHT [38]. MAHT is related to increases in *sympathetic nerve activity* and *insulin resistance* [39]. Significantly higher *resistin* levels have been found in individuals with MAHT compared to normotensive ones [40-41]. Human resistin is an inflammatory mediator and a biomarker of CV diseases, especially in atherosclerosis and heart failure [42].

4. Prevalence

A major issue concerns the prevalence of MAHT. Although there are no definitive data, the available information is disturbing [5]. There is increasing evidence that the prevalence of WC-AHT and of MAHT is significant. MAHT requires treatment, while WC-AHT does not. Since neither of these conditions can be diagnosed by office BP measurements alone, over-treatment is possible for WC-AHT and under-treatment for MAHT -unless HBPM or ABPM is used [43].

MAHT is a relatively common phenomenon, whose prevalence varies from *8%-45%,* due to the heterogeneity of the study populations [17, 44]. Data obtained in several cross-sectional studies have demonstrated large differences in the prevalence of MAHT: prevalence rates from *8%-49%* [11, 44-48].

MAHT is reported to be seen in about *10%–20%* of the general populations [8, 28]. While the prevalence of MAHT is not entirely clear, the „syndrome" may be present in as many as 10% of normotensive or prehypertensive individuals [49]. In a study of 319 clinically normotensive volunteers, all of whom had 5 clinic measurements and 12-hour daytime ABPM, authors found that *23%* had MAHT, defined as a daytime BP >135/85 mmHg. In the Cornell Worksite study, *13.5%* of 267 men had MAHT, defined as a *daytime ambulatory dBP >85 mmHg and a clinic BP <85 mmHg* [5]. Prevalence of MAHT in adults is *at least 10%* [50]. MAHT was present in *15%* of participants who had BP measured in the workplace and by ABPM [26]. MAHT is more frequently found in prehypertensive individuals. Recent study showed a MAHT prevalence of 8.1%. Although no definitive data are available, MAHT prevalence has been estimated to be *10%–38%,* depending on the diagnostic criteria used to identify this condition and the characteristics of the population examined. MAHT is prevalent and *may be even more so*: as HBPM becomes more popular, the detection MAHT will increase [7].

Two population-based studies are more likely to reflect unbiased estimates of MAHT prevalence. In the Pressione Arteriose Monitorate E Loro Associazioni (PAMELA) population of 3200 Italians, who had clinic visits and ABPM, *9%* had MAHT ("reverse WC-AHT"). Individuals with treated AHT were excluded from this analysis [11]. In the cohort of elderly men prospectively surveyed in the Uppsala Longitudinal Study of Adult Men, MAHT prevalence was *14%* [7, 45].

In a study, conducted in patients consecutively attending an academic family medicine clinic, 34.6% had sBP readings and 23.8% diastolic pressures, which were lower during the clinic visits than at home. The high percentage of patients with *"home hypertension"* may simply be related to the time of BP measurement in relation to the time taking the medications [11]. Studies have shown the prevalence of MAHT to range from *10% to 47%* of subjects considered normotensive by conventional office BP measurements [5, 18, 25. 51]. MAHT prevalence also depends on the technique used to measure out-of-office BP. Likewise, MAHT was detected in *10.6%* of subjects by HBPM and in *11.4%* of subjects by ABPM [18].

An extrapolation to the national population of Spain was made to estimate the absolute number of hypertensive subjects in the 4 BP groups at a Spanish population level, assuming universality of ABPM performance in the 8 million AHT patients, treated in outpatient clinics in Spain: Approximately *1.9 million* patients were *clinically controlled*, ≈1.5 of whom were controlled by both methods, and ≈0.4 million were patients whose BP control was overestimated using clinical measurements at the office. Of the *6.1 million* subjects with *clinically uncontrolled* AHT, only 3.4 million were uncontrolled when ABPM was used, because the rest were false-negatives or "office resistant," and their BP control was, thus, underestimated at the office [12]. A recent analysis was published of baseline data from the African American Study of Kidney (AASK) Disease Cohort Study in subjects with controlled clinic BP (<140/90 mmHg). MAHT was defined by elevated daytime (≥135/85 mmHg) or elevated nighttime (≥120/70 mmHg) ABPM in those with controlled clinic BP (<140/90 mmHg). Of the 61% of participants with controlled office BP, *70% had MAHT* [3]. Using ABPM, authors discovered that *25%* of the *prehypertensive* subjects had MAHT in one study, and *20%* in the other [17]. MAHT is common and should be considered in individuals with a normal resting office BP but a *hypertensive response to exercise*. This observation may help to explain the increased risk associated with a hypertensive response to exercise [52].

In the study of Rodrigues et al., MAHT was observed in *13.6%* out of 103 clinical *normotensive* patients with *type 1 DM*; 23% of subjects with clinical normotension had *nocturnal* MAHT. High normal BP values during the night (thus, even within the normotensive range), were linked to altered renal hemodynamic parameters, albuminuria and autonomic dysfunction in patients with type 1 DM [44]. In normotensive *type 2 DM* patients, the prevalence of MAHT has been estimated between *18% and 47%* [44]. The recent studies have revealed the prevalence of MAHT in the type 2 diabetic patients from *30% to 47%* [31].

MAHT is frequent (28.9%) in population with a documented *vascular disease* under medication, with no prior history of AHT. The screening of MAHT in these patients is necessary. The prehypertensive rank seems to be a good predictor of MAHT [53]. Among 980 patients with *CKD,* identified in 6 studies, the overall prevalence of MAHT was *8.3%* and of WC-AHT was 18.3%. *More alarming, 40.4% of patients who had CKD and were thought to have normotension (or adequately treated AHT), in fact had high BP at home.* Also 30.0% of patients who had CKD and were thought to have AHT had normal BP at home [54]. Using ABPM, Hayder and colleagues identified MAHT in *15%* of 241 kidney transplant recipients [55]. MAHT was found in *8%-9% of children* evaluated at two large AHT centers. MAHT predisposed to the progress toward sustained AHT and LVH, especially in children with parental history of AHT [56]. *Children* with MAHT had significantly greater LV mass in comparison with confirmed *normotensive* subjects. LV mass indices in children with MAHT were similar on average to AHT patients, findings which resemble those in adults. It suggests that MAHT patients have more extensive structural cardiac abnormalities than confirmed normotensives [57]. Insufficient BP control („masked effect“, sometimes called MAHT) was found in many AHT patients. Office resistance (WC-AHT) and isolated office control (MAHT) are not usually reported, but are common in daily practice [12]. MAHT was initially regarded as rare, but was recently found to be present, to some extent, in as many as *1/3 of the hypertensive population* [6, 58, 59]. In the AASK study, despite intensive drug treatment to lower BP, *42%* of the subjects had MAHT [3, 20].

5. Classification

According to many authors, there are basically two types of MAHT:

1) MAHT in *general population* (*10-15%, which makes hundred millions in the world*) in people with normal office BP, but elevated out-of-office BP (e.g. at workplace).
2) The other type of MAHT occurs in *≈30%* of patients with *sustained AHT*, who have diagnosed AHT and apparently well-controlled BP (by means of treatment), i.e. normal office BP, but not normal BP all day long (e.g. BP is uncontrolled, mostly in the morning and/or in the night).

Other doctors believe that only the first type is MAHT, while the second is only *"insufficiently efficient antihypertensive therapy," "inadequate AHT control" or "masking effect."* This is probably the better nomenclature. Whatever the name, insufficient BP control is crucial to recognize. Both physicians and patients are not enough aware of this fact, as judged by insufficient usage of long-acting antihypertensives, by the absence of the antihypertensive drug dose in the evening (or at night), by insufficient ABPM and HBPM in everyday practice, as well as by the results of ABPM and HBPM studies.

Classification of MAHT into subtypes, according to BP circadian cycle (*morning* hypertension, *daytime* hypertension, and *night-time* hypertension, regardless of the presence of antihypertensive treatment) has been recently proposed as the subtypes may reflect different pathogenetic mechanisms [7]. An exaggerated increase in sympathetic activity at the end of the night-time rest, excessive alcohol consumption, or short-acting antihypertensive drugs may have a role in *morning hypertension* ("morning BP surge"), while smoking habit, intense exercise, mental stress, heavy meals, excessive alcohol intake and their combination may give raise to *daytime hypertension*. Moreover, all conditions associated with a blunted BP fall at night (such as: DM, sleep apnea, autonomic failure, renal dysfunction and high Na^+ intake in salt-sensitive individuals) may determine *nocturnal hypertension* [7].

A. Clinical Relevance – MAHT and Progression to Sustained AHT

MAHT has been related to an increased risk of *sustained AHT* and *CV morbidity* [18, 45, 48, 51, 60-63]. MAHT in youth can be a precursor to the development of sustained AHT (24). MAHT predisposed to the development of sustained AHT and LVH, especially in children with parental history of AHT [56]. MAHT has been linked with an *increased CV risk.* A 3-year follow-up study of children diagnosed in whom MAHT was diagnosed has shown that *≈50% of them had persistent elevated ABPM* or progressed to clinical MAHT 3 years later [64, 65]. It is believed that MAHT is not a benign condition, because about half of people with MAHT develop sustained AHT over a 10-year follow-up, compared with 20% of ''true normotensive'' subjects [51, 66].

B. Clinical Relevance – MAHT and Hypertensive TOD

MAHT is associated with hypertensive TOD [8, 11, 17, 46]. Patients with MAHT have more extensive hypertensive TOD in comparison with true normotensive subjects. The first study to look at this issue was published in *1999.* It revealed that the MAHT group had *LV mass* and *carotid atherosclerosis* that were greater than that of true normotensive subjects and that were similar to true AHT patients [5]. The pioneering paper was published by Liu and colleagues, showing that 61 individuals recruited from work sites with office normotension and daytime ambulatory sBP or dBP ≥140/90 mmHg had a more pronounced cardiac and vascular involvement, as compared to 234 sustained normotensives. Since then, a few studies have addressed the relationship between MAHT and LV structural changes [7, 46]. MAHT patients, diagnosed by both ABPM and HBPM, had a greater *LVMI* than *normotensive* subjects [8]. MAHT patients have increased *LV mass* than *normotensive* subjects. Similarly, patients with MAHT are more likely to have *thickening of CCA-IMT.* Moreover, MAHT patients showed a TOD involvement similar to that of sustained AHT. A recent prospective study of Pierdomenico et al. demonstrated that among *prehypertensive* individuals, those with MAHT were at higher CV risk than those without MAHT [17].

Electrocardiographic LVH was found to be independently correlated to MAHT [7, 19]. In the PAMELA population, patients with MAHT had a prevalence of *echocardiographic LVH* that was much greater than that of *normotensive* subjects [6]. In the PAMELA study, *LVMI* in WC-AHT was increased similarly to that in MAHT (participants with WC-AHT were older than those in the MAHT group) [8]. Cuspidi and coworkers reported in an *updated 2012 overview* that increased LV mass was more frequently found in MAHT patients compared to non- MAHT counterparts, although a wide range of values was present among the reports (7%–66%). Moreover, *LVH prevalence was approximately 3-fold higher (29%) in MAHT as compared with non-MAHT subjects (9%)* [7].

MAHT –defined as usually (normal office BP, but raised BP at home or on ABPM)- is lined to *raised risk of vascular events.* It has been assumed to be due to the fact that *mean BP is higher than was recorded in the doctor's office*. In fact, increased vascular risk is likely to be due, at least in part, to variability in BP, MAHT being only one manifestation of variability [67]. Patients with MAHT have *elevated large artery stiffness* and enhanced plasma levels of components known to promote endothelial dysfunction [40, 68, 69]. In the studies of clinic outpatients, MAHT -defined by HBPM- has also been related to a risk of increased *carotid intima-media thickness (CIMT)* [68] and CV events [8, 48].

Recently, *nocturnal* MAHT was found in 30% in a cohort of clinical *normotensive type 2 DM* patients and it was accompanied by *increased arterial stiffness* and *higher central BP* (44). MAHT, determined by ABPM, was associated with a *higher serum glucose level* and *UAR,* but MAHT defined by HBPM was not. MAHT was related to a higher *glycemia,* although the average age was lower in the MAHT group versus the other hypertensive groups. Glucose-related sympathetic nerve overactivity (raised daytime BP), and decreased Na^+ excretion capacity is needed to compensate during night-time (nocturnal AHT) [8]. Furthermore, MAHT defined by ABPM was associated with a high *glucose* level and urinary albumin-creatinine ratio at a relatively younger age [8, 64].

In comparison with *normotensives,* MAHT patients had *higher urinary albumin-creatinine ratio, thicker LV wall* and preclinical *impairment of LV diastolic function* (44). MAHT patients (defined as office BP ≤140/90 mmHg and 24-hour ambulatory BP ≥130/80 mmHg) had a *higher serum glucose level* (126 versus 96 mg/dL, P=0.001) and *urinary albumin-creatinine ratio* (38.0 versus 7.5 mg/gCr, P<0.001) than the *normotensive* participants; however, these relationships were not observed when the authors defined groups using HBPM (≥135/85 mmHg) [8].

Although *HBPM* is predictive of MAHT defined by ABPM, it is usually measured in a *sitting position at rest,* while ambulatory BP can be measured under a variety of conditions (including *physical activity* or resting /sleeping in a *supine position*). Therefore, depending on exactly what one is trying to measure, HBPM may not be an adequate substitute for 24-hour ABPM. Nocturnal AHT, defined by ABPM among participants with HBPM <135/85 mmHg, was linked to *increased LV mass* and *CIMT.* However, MAHT defined by HBPM has also been reported to be associated with increased CIMT, pulse wave velocity, and risk of CV events in clinic outpatients [8].

In a subset of patients with *type 1 DM,* who are *normotensive* at the office, the prevalence of MAHT and nocturnal MAHT is high. Night sBP and dBP (rather than nocturnal dipping BP pattern or the others BP parameters analyzed), were the most important factor related to *diabetic retinopathy.* ABPM is useful as an additional tool in the periodical evaluation of type 1 DM patients, especially those with normal BP at the office. ABPM identifies more accurately the patients at elevated risk for diabetic retinopathy [44].

In the study of Mitsnefes and coworkers, multivariable analysis demonstrated that MAHT (OR 4.1) and confirmed AHT (OR 4.3) were the strongest independent predictors of *LVH in children with CKD.* Thus, casual BP measurements alone are insufficient to predict the presence of LVH. The high prevalence of MAHT and its interrelation with LVH supports the usefulness early echocardiography and ABPM to appraise CV risk in children with CKD [70].

Indeed, in *treated* AHT patients, insufficient BP control (sometimes called MAHT or -better- masking effect) results in worse outcome. For example, a total of 332 outpatients with chronically treated essential AHT were enrolled in the study of Tomiyama et al. Participants were classified into 4 groups according to office (<140/90 or ≥140/90 mmHg) and daytime ambulatory (<135/85 or ≥135/85 mmHg) BP levels; i.e., *controlled* AHT (low both office and ambulatory BP), *WC-AHT* (high office but low ambulatory BP), *MAHT* (low office but high ambulatory BP), and *sustained* AHT (high both office and ambulatory BP). *LV mass index (LVMI), maximal CIMT* and *urinary albumin level* in MAHT were significantly higher than in controlled AHT and WC-AHT, and were similar to those in sustained AHT. Multivariate regression analyses showed that MAHT was one of the independent determinants of LVH, carotid atherosclerosis, and albuminuria. Therefore, MAHT is connected to *advanced TOD* in *treated* hypertensive patients [71].

C. Clinical Relevance – MAHT and Comorbidity

MAHT is linked with CV events [8, 45, 62]. An early study provided the evidence that MAHT amplifies incidence of CV events. In a population-based cohort of 578 untreated 70-year-old men, it was found that both MAHT and sustained AHT were *independent predictors of CV events (coronary fatal and nonfatal coronary events, stroke and peripheral vascular deaths),* the relative risk (RR) being 2.77 and 2.94, respectively. These data support the view that *important prognostic information is missed when BP is only measured in the clinical setting* [7, 45].

MAHT is associated with CKD progression and with increased CV deaths in patients with or without normal kidney function [48, 54, 72, 73]. ABPM is recommended for kidney transplant patients to screen and diagnose AHT post–kidney transplantation, to identify MAHT and disturbances in day-night BP patterns, and to eliminate the false-positive diagnosis of AHT due to the white coat effect. When ABPM is not readily available, self-measured BP is the best substitute. ABPM performed during the first year following transplantation will assist in achieving these targets and will help to identify MAHT and disturbances in the day-night BP pattern [14].

Out of 130 newly diagnosed OSA patients, 31.5% were normotensive, *30.0% had MAHT*, 3.1% WC-AHT and 35.4% AHT. Important differences were established between normotensive, MAHT and hypertensive participants in terms of carotid IMT and LVMI. A clinic sBP >125 and a dBP >83 mmHg led to a RR of 2.7 and a 90% positive predictive value for having MAHT. *MAHT is frequently underestimated in OSA and is nearly always present when office BP is >125/83 mmHg* [21]. MAHT is related to *increases in sympathetic nerve activity* and *insulin resistance*, which is important, both for pathophysiology and comorbidity evaluation [39].

Data of Ishikawa et al. support previous reports, which have revealed a correlation between MAHT and *increased glucose levels* or *presence of DM* [8]. Marchesi et al. found link of MAHT in type 2 DM patients with remodeling of LV characterized by increased myocardial mass and impairment of diastolic functions [74].

AHT is the major source of AF and MAHT causes morbidity and mortality close to sustained AHT. Therefore, MAHT is probably capable of causing almost all what AHT does, e.g. AF. Certain factors are recognized causes of both AF and MAHT, e.g. excessive alcohol consumption; stress (both mental and physical); high heart rate; OSA. Hence, MAHT may be another reason to explain lone AF, which is not always so „lonely". In other words, some lone AFs may well be the consequence of MAHT. It seems logical (and worth checking) to perform 24h ABPM in patients with lone AF, at least if they have prehypertension [75].

D. Clinical Relevance –Prognosis

According to currently available medical literature, MAHT is prevalent, important for prognosis, associated with subclinical damages and treatable form of AHT, but insufficiently recognized entity. Part of prognosis is determined by hypertensive TOD, as aforementioned. The first study to look at TOD in MAHT was published in 1999. It showed that the MAHT group had LV mass and carotid atherosclerosis which were greater than that of true normotensive subjects and which were similar to true AHT subjects. The LVMI was 73 g/m^2

in the true normotensive individuals, 86 g/m^2 in the MAHT subjects, and 90 g/m^2 in the true AHT patients. Carotid plaque was present in 15% of true normotensives and in 28% of both the MAHT and true AHT patients [46]. MAHT patients (with normal BP in the physician's office but high BP during daily life) were found to have a higher risk of CV events. For clinicians, the danger lies in underestimating the patient's risk of CV events and, thus, undertreating the AHT. Preliminary data on MAHT show that the rates of end-organ damage and CV events could be even slightly higher in patients with MAHT than in patients with sustained AHT [76].

In the PAMELA study, the increment in the risk of developing sustained AHT in WC-AHT and MAHT remained substantially unaltered when calculations excluded subjects reporting an antihypertensive drug assumption, and its size was similar in untreated and treated individuals.

Interestingly, because subjects with WC-AHT and MAHT showed a somewhat attenuated rise in dBP, the more pronounced increase was even more evident for pulse pressure. This could mean that their greater rate of progression to sustained AHT depends at least in part to a more pronounced stiffening of the large arteries. BP variability may be a precursor of a steady hypertensive state [51].

Compared with a true normotensive condition, the greater risk of new-onset *sustained AHT* exhibited by WC-AHT and MAHT is by no means marginal, because the age- and sex-adjusted risks were almost *doubled* and more than *tripled* when these conditions were diagnosed, respectively, by office and HBPM / ABPM. Because the incidence of CV fatal and nonfatal events and mortality is greater in the presence of sustained AHT than when only the in-office or out-of-office BP value is increased, *these results provide a strong argument against the clinical "innocence" of these conditions, supporting their adverse long-term prognostic significance instead* [51].

In a cohort of 4939 treated *hypertensive* patients, in a multivariable model with patients having controlled AHT (normal both home and office BP) as the referent, the hazard ratio of CV events was 1.96 in patients with uncontrolled AHT (high BP by both measurement methods), *2.06* in patients with normal office BP and elevated home BP, and 1.18 in patients with elevated office BP and normal home BP [25].

In a study of 340 patients with controlled AHT (responders, with clinic BP <140/90 mmHg and daytime BP <135/85 mmHg), 126 with MAHT (clinic BP <140/90 mmHg and daytime BP >135 or 85 mmHg), 146 with false resistant (WC-AHT) (clinic BP ≥140 or 90 mmHg and daytime BP <135/85 mmHg), and 130 with true resistant AHT (non-responders, with office BP ≥140 or 90 mmHg and daytime BP >135 or 85 mmHg). During 5 years follow-up period, the event-rate per 100 patient-years was 0.87, *2.42,* 1.2, and 4.1 in responders, *MAHT,* false resistant and true resistant AHT, respectively. Patients with MAHT are at higher risk than those with responder AHT, and that those with false resistant AHT are at lower risk than those with true resistant AHT. ABPM should be performed in treated AHT patients to obtain a better prognostic stratification [77].

Several, but not all of the previous studies, have indeed suggested that MAHT may be related to the increased CV risk that is close to that of sustained AHT [78]. Three meta-analyses have evaluated the prognostic significance of MAHT and WC-AHT using ABPM. One involved participants from four populations, one also included *hypertensive* patients from primary or specialist care and the other investigated initially *untreated* individuals. The 3 meta-analyses reported similar results. *MAHT* and sustained AHT showed a *significantly higher CV risk than normotension*, even after adjustment for other traditional risk factors, whereas the risk associated with WC-AHT was not significantly different from that of normotension [61, 63, 78, 79]. When treated participants were excluded from the analyses, similar results were obtained as in the total study population [62, 78, 80].

In previous general population–based studies, as well as in the two meta-analyses, the increased CV risk in MAHT usually remained significant after adjustment for traditional CV risk factors, and further adjustment for office BP did not substantially change the results [61-63, 78, 80]. At baseline, MAHT patients had a higher frequency of conventional CV risk factors. The risk of all-cause mortality was higher in MAHT than in normotension after adjustment for age, sex and office BP. MAHT, however, lost its predictive significance in Cox models adjusted for home BP or concomitant other CV risk factors. Thus, MAHT patients had higher age-adjusted CV risk than normotensive individuals when the diagnosis was based on HBPM in a nationwide general population. Because both MAHT and WC-AHT patients had intermediate BP levels and concomitant other CV risk factors, their overall CV risk laid between that of normotensive individuals and that of sustained AHT patients. MAHT also had a higher risk of all-cause mortality after adjustment for age, sex and office BP. However, MAHT was not an independent predictor of CV risk or all-cause mortality when concomitant other risk factors or baseline home BP levels were taken into account [78].

Ohasama study was the first to report that MAHT is related to increased CV risk among women and treated subjects, irrespective of the number of risk factors or CV complications. Importantly, even among subjects with a low CV risk profile, MAHT is linked to a significantly greater risk of stroke and CV mortality [62]. Ohasama results suggest that 16 truly high-risk subjects of every 100 persons without antihypertensive medication may not be identified under conventional casual BP measurements, but could be detected using ABPM. Also, 18 truly uncontrolled patients out of every 100 patients under antihypertensive medication may not be identified under casual BP measurements, but could be detected using ABPM. Unless individuals with MAHT are identified, they will remain untreated or inadequately controlled and might experience CV complications and TOD, resulting in poor quality of life. Unnecessary medical costs also will be incurred. This in turn suggests the possibility that detection and management of AHT -based on ABPM- could improve prognosis for at-risk populations [62].

MAHT patients had a higher ambulatory pulse rate than normotensive subjects, were more obese, and were more than twice as likely to have a parental history of AHT. These 3 characteristics, alone or in combination, predict the development of AHT and increase CV risk later in life. Tachycardia and high BMI are usually accompanied by stimulation of the sympathetic nervous system, which (together with the raised daytime BP and obesity) might underlie the complicating LVH in youth with MAHT, even before they proceed to sustained AHT (64). Physicians should not lightly decide to dismiss treatment in patients with WC-AHT. Normal clinic BP values should not be taken as a guarantee that there is no increase in risk, because of the possibility of an increase in out-of-office BP. This implies that out-of-office BP values should be more frequently recorded than is recommended by current guidelines [81].

Neither MAHT nor WC-AHT was an independent predictor of CV risk or all-cause mortality, when concomitant other risk factors or baseline home BP levels were taken into account. Home BP level, along with other traditional risk factors, may be enough to stratify

CV risk [78]. Children with WC-AHT and MAHT require regular follow-up as they are at risk of sustained AHT [82, 83].

Hermida's et al. had performed a study on the *prognostic value of ABPM,* using highly reproducible 48h ABPM and wrist actigraphy, in a relatively large cohort of subjects with baseline BP ranging from normotension to AHT. Results reveal the higher prognostic value of CV events for ABPM than clinic BP measurements, as documented in previous studies, mainly when asleep BP is used for classification and CV risk assessment. Such findings, in agreement with most cross-sectional studies on this topic, indicate that the *asleep sBP mean best predicted CV events* in a Cox proportional-hazard model adjusted by relevant confounding variables. *Awake BP, however, was not a significant predictor of CV outcome in a fully adjusted model also including asleep BP mean.* There might be only two possible groups of subjects when using BP measurements for CV risk assessment: Those with either normal asleep BP or elevated asleep BP, independently of the level of either clinic or awake BP measurements. Some studies, following the published recommendation of international guidelines, classified subjects into the classes of normotension, isolated-office AHT, MAHT, and sustained AHT by comparing clinic with awake BP mean. While each of these two BP measurements, as virtually any parameter derived from conventional, HBPM, or ABPM, are to some extent individually correlated with CV risk, none of them provide any valuable added prognostic information when the asleep BP is used as a confounding variable for survival analyses [83].

The use for classification of the 24-hour BP mean, instead of awake BP, in a minority of reports does not seem to be adequate either. First, current guidelines recommend the preferable use of awake and asleep BP means, instead of the 24-hour mean, for diagnosis of AHT; second, subjects with exactly the same 24-hour BP mean might have a BP pattern ranging from extreme-dipping to rising (asleep BP above awake BP mean), and would thus have markedly different CV risk [83].

Apart from the marked difference in CVD risk assessment when using awake or asleep BP means for comparison with clinic BP, findings of Hermida and coworkers indicate the reported information on the prevalence of the resulting four categories, and thus on the real clinical dimension of MAHT and isolated-office AHT, is surely incorrect. For example, 58.2% of subjects who should be labeled as MAHT based on their elevated asleep BP have been so far classified as normotensive (based on normal awake BP) and thus mistakenly included in the reference group for evaluating CV risk of other categories; 38.2% of subjects with normal asleep BP and thus at low CV risk have been always classified as MAHT [83]. Encouragingly, BP control based on ABPM was more than twice as good as control based on conventional measurement [12].

6. Screening for MAHT

A. Who Should Be Screened for MAHT?

What should arouse suspicion of MAHT and motivate physicians to initiate a further work-up [6]? The answer is logical - persons at risk for MAHT should undergo screening for MAHT. Admittedly, prospective studies have not proved cost-effectiveness of this approach, yet. Individuals with normal office BP in whom MAHT should be searched for are the following:

- young
- male
- with unfavorable lifestyle (smoking, drinking)
- obese
- with DM
- with kidney disease (proteinuria)
- with OSA
- with high-normal office BP
- with transiently elevated BP
- with a hypertensive response to exercise
- hyper-reactive to standing
- at high CV risk
- with echocardiographic LVH
- with the presence of *inappropriate* TOD (such as LVH or microalbuminuria) or office BP levels [3, 6, 10, 20-23, 29, 30, 44, 46, 47, 84-86].

ABPM for those at risk for MAHT needs to be incorporated into guidelines [20].

B. How to Screen for MAHT?

BP is a very labile hemodynamic parameter; it varies from heartbeat to heartbeat, from morning to evening, from winter to summer, from sleeping to awake, and from sitting to standing. The same holds true for any other CV hemodynamic parameter such as heart rate, cardiac output, LV ejection fraction or pulmonary wedge pressure [6].

BP measured in the physician's office has long been used to diagnose AHT and evaluate treatment efficacy. However, the correlation between BP level and TOD, CV risk, and long-term prognosis is greater for ABPM than clinical BP measurements [83]. The combined use of office and out-of-office BP has allowed a more accurate classification of subjects. Office hypertensive patients have been subdivided into sustained AHT and WC-AHT (i.e. elevated office BP, but normal out-of-office BP). Similarly, office normotensive individuals have been subdivided into normotensives and MAHT (i.e. elevated out-of-office BP, despite a normal office BP) [78].

C. Both ABPM and HBPM Are Good to Detect MAHT

The use of HBPM on a regular basis should be considered for patients with AHT, particularly those with:

- DM (Grade D);
- CKD (Grade C);

- Suspected nonadherence (Grade D);
- Demonstrated white coat effect (Grade C);
- *BP controlled in the office, but not at home (MAHT)* (Grade C) [87].

ABPM and HBPM allow two specific clinical conditions to be diagnosed, namely WC-AHT (isolated clinic AHT), characterized by higher office BP with normal ambulatory BP values, and MAHT, characterized by normal office BP with high ambulatory BP values [88]. The best method for identifying MAHT is still debated. Systematic use of *HBPM* might represent a *less expensive* and *more repeatable* alternative to ABPM. This approach, however, has the limitation to miss elevated BP periods during working or during night-time hours [7].

There are the studies investigating MAHT prognosis, which suggest that the predictive value of MAHT is not affected by the methods used for out-of-office BP determination. This was also the case for MAHT association with subclinical organ damage (e.g., LVH) [7].

Similar proportions of subjects with MAHT are detected by ABPM and HBPM. Although disagreement in the diagnosis between the two methods is not uncommon, in the majority of these cases, the deviation of the diagnostic BP above the threshold in not clinically important. Both ABPM and HBPM appear to be appropriate methods for the detection of MAHT [89].

There are fewer prospective studies using HBPM, and only two that have *compared ABPM with self-BP monitoring (the Ohasama and PAMELA studies).* Both of these studies found that *the two methods had similar predictive value for future CV events* [1].

The use of HBPM as an adjunct to office BP measurements has been recommended by several national and international guidelines for the management of AHT, including the European Society of Hypertension (ESH), the American Society of Hypertension (ASH), the American Heart Association (AHA), the British Hypertension Society, the Japanese Hypertension Society, the World Health Organization– International Society of Hypertension, and the Joint National Committee on Prevention, Detection, Evaluation, and Treatment of High Blood Pressure (JNC 7) [49, 90-97]. HBPM and ABPM detect a similar, but not an identical, group of MAHT individuals. Their agreement in the diagnosis of MAHT is only moderate. The results of Hänninen et al. suggest that HBPM measurement can be used to diagnose MAHT, but this diagnosis is not analogous with that made with ABPM [98].

D. ABPM May Be Better to Detect MAHT, as Compared to HBPM

Even in treated AHT patients, a high out of-office BP is a marker for increased risk. Attributable to its inherent variability, using a small number of readings yields poor reproducibility for the BP level. *By increasing the number of readings used to calculate the average, both self and 24-hour ABPM give much better estimates of the average.* In one study, home BP was the most reproducible (lowest standard deviation of the differences between sets of measurements: 6.9/4.7 mmHg for sBP and dBP for self-BP, 8.3/5.6 mmHg for ambulatory BP, and 11.0/6.6 mmHg for office BP) [1].

Some authors believe that the ability of HBPM to identify those with MAHT or WC-AHT defined by 24-hour ABPM is poor, and we may need to perform ABPM for participants with borderline BP levels [8]. *MAHT was detected in 10.6% of subjects by HBPM and in 11.4% of subjects by ABPM.* Although both methods can be used to make this diagnosis, ABPM is more likely to note MAHT (particularly with inclusion of nocturnal cutoff values) [18]. BP measured over 24 hours by an *ABPM is the best method* for estimating an individual's CV risk related to AHT. This has been established in a large number of prospective cohort studies, most of which have shown that the office BP has negligible prospective value if the 24-hour BP is known [1].

Current guidelines define normotension and "sustained" AHT as a consistently normal or elevated BP, respectively, on both clinic and ambulatory measurements. Discrepancies between the two measurements have been defined as isolated-office AHT and MAHT. The same guidelines recommend the use of separate threshold values for daytime and nighttime BP means for diagnosis of AHT based on ABPM. However, classification of subjects into isolated-office and MAHT has most frequently relied, as suggested in the guidelines themselves, on comparison of clinic and awake BP mean, disregarding entirely the asleep BP mean otherwise used to define AHT. Past studies have mostly, but not consistently, found that CV risk does not differ significantly between WC-AHT and normotension, but is significantly higher in MAHT and sustained AHT than in normotension. A major limitation of all these previous studies is that, by classifying subjects from comparison of clinic and ambulatory awake or even 24-hour BP measurements, each of the four resulting categories could include individuals with normal and elevated asleep BP, and thus at a markedly different CV risk. This appears to be clinically relevant, because a growing number of studies have concluded that the nighttime BP mean is a better predictor of CV risk than the awake or 24-hour BP means. The Monitorización Ambulatoria para Predicción de Eventos Cardiovasculares (MAPEC), (i.e., Ambulatory BP Monitoring for Prediction of Cardiovascular Events) study was specifically designed to investigate prospectively whether specific changes in the circadian BP profile during follow-up results in reduced CV risk. It shows the higher prognostic value of CV events for ABPM than clinic BP measurements, as documented in previous studies, mainly when asleep BP is used for classification and CV risk assessment [83].

In principle, one would expect that 24-hour ABPM would give a better prediction of risk because there are *important aspects of the circadian profile of BP that are detected by ambulatory recordings, but not by self/home BP measurements.* These include: *BP variability, the morning surge of BP, nocturnal BP and the related measures of dipping* [1].

HBPM, although useful in assessing BP control in clinical practice, is not as informative as ABPM and cannot provide nocturnal pressures. The common patterns of ABPM include WC-AHT, white-coat effect, systo-diastolic AHT, (isolated) systolic AHT, (isolated) diastolic AHT, nocturnal dipping and nondipping, reverse dipping, extreme dipping, siesta dipping, isolated nocturnal AHT, the morning surge, MAHT and ambulatory hypotension [50].

MAHT defined by ABPM was associated with increased glucose level and urinary albumin-creatinine excretion ratio. MAHT defined by HBPM may not have the same ability to predict CV risk factors and hypertensive TOD as MAHT defined by ABPM [8]. BP reductions of ≈20% during sleep relative to the awake period are observed in most people undergoing 24-hour ABPM. However, a substantial minority of AHT patients have a lesser decline in nocturnal BP. A reduced or absent decline in sleep BP, also referred to as a nondipping pattern, is more prevalent as people age, in African-Americans, and in postmenopausal women (especially if of African-American origin). There is consistent evidence that the absence of a BP decline during sleep is related to the increased TOD including LVH, albuminuria, and microvascular disease of the brain [49].

Consequently, asleep BP is very important. MAHT is an emerging clinical entity predisposing to subclinical organ damage and to increased CV risk [78]. The best way to diagnose MAHT is to use ABPM, because sleep-time BP can not be measured otherwise noninvasively. Evidence for the circadian periodicity of BP being synchronized with the sleep–wake cycle also comes from observations in shift workers. For example, it is known that a complete and nearly immediate reversal of the BP rhythm occurs on the first occasion of a session of night shifts compared to daytime work hours. As a result of the shift in work schedules, the peak sBP in night workers is recorded at about 11 p.m. and the dBP peaks at about 10 p.m. [49, 99, 100].

MAHT, particularly *nocturnal* BP control, may account for the disappointing results from the AASK study where despite excellent in-office BP control there was still progression of kidney disease. These studies indicate that MAHT is difficult to recognize by usual BP monitoring in the office [3]. Nocturnal AHT is commonly found in patients with type 2 DM and clinic BP levels below the currently recommended diagnostic threshold and treatment goal. Identification of patients with masked nocturnal AHT has the potential to improve risk stratification as these patients had increased arterial stiffness and higher central BP [85]. Defining normal ambulatory BP according to daytime (awake state) measurements alone may misclassify $\geq$4% of the patients as controlled, whereas, in fact, their 24-hour BP is abnormal. To be valid, the *daytime* BP average used to judge ambulatory BP normality must only include measurements taken in the *awake* state. Had values recorded during daytime napping (namely, siesta) been included with the awake measurements, they would falsely lower these averages, thus erroneously presenting high rates of daytime ambulatory BP control. It was the point with the adequate title: "Is siesta *masking masked* hypertension?" [101].

A *morning surge* is defined as *arise in BP>55 mmHg from the lowest night-time reading.* CV events, such as acute myocardial infarction (AMI), ischemia and stroke, are more frequent in the morning hours soon after waking than at other times of day. Circadian variations in biochemical and physiological parameters help to explain the link between acute CV events and the early morning BP surge. In older hypertensive subjects with a morning surge the risk of stroke is increased almost threefold [50]. Early morning BP surge is important.

A rapid rise in both BP and heart rate often occurs in the morning upon awakening. Epidemiologic studies have shown that coinciding with this early morning BP surge period, there is an increase in the rates of CV events including sudden death, AMI, and stroke. Non-hemodynamic factors (including plaque vulnerability and increased coagulability) contribute to the early morning prothrombotic state that may lead to some of these events [49].

Studies have consistently revealed that AMI is more prevalent between 6 a.m. and noon than at other times of the day or night. Moreover, it is verified that the incidence of subarachnoid hemorrhage, ischemic stroke, hemorrhagic stroke, and transient ischemic attacks is also highest in the first few hours after awakening. Evidence for a link between the morning surge in BP and cerebrovascular damage comes from a study conducted in elderly Japanese AHT patients by Kario et al. *Using ABPM, the extent of the early-morning BP surge was defined as the difference between the average sBP during the 2 hours after awakening minus the average sBP during the 1 hour that included the lowest sleeping sBP.* The 519 patients studied were divided into two groups according to deciles of the surge. In the group of patients which had a surge of >55 mmHg (top decile), the risk of multiple lacunar infarctions was approximately two-fold higher -after matching for age and the 24-hour BP- compared to the non-surge patients (average morning sBP increase of 9 mmHg). The authors concluded that future randomized trials should investigate the ability of antihypertensive agents to suppress the morning BP surge and affect outcomes. Similarly, Li et al. reported that while accounting for the night-to-day BP ratio, the 24-hour BP level, and other covariates, a morning surge in BP exceeding the 90th percentile was a significant and independent predictor of mortality and CV events. One approach for this well-described issue is to tailor treatment that remains highly effective for all 24 hours of the dosing period, to provide target-organ protection. Hence, this is one area – the early morning BP – that is much easier to assess with out-of-office monitoring than in the clinic, as it is impractical and complicated to obtain multiple readings at different times of the day (and dosing interval) in the ambulatory medical care environment [49, 102-107].

Studies have shown that BP measured over 24 hours by ABPM is the most robust method to predict CV risk related to AHT [49, 73, 108]. Studied retrospectively, Ben-Dov and coauthors found WC-AHT and the masking phenomenon to be at least reasonably reproducible in real-life ABPM practice [109]. MAHT appears to have only moderate reproducibility, favoring the hypothesis that office BP measurements may systematically fail to identify subjects who should be treated as hypertensive [49]. *Exercise brachial sBP* predicted the presence of MAHT independent from all resting hemodynamic variables, and *if >190mmHg, identified MAHT with 97% specificity* ($p < 0.001$). Thus, MAHT can be identified ("*unmasked*") in untreated individuals from low intensity exercise brachial sBP. *Exercise BP testing may be indicated in individuals with borderline raised clinic brachial sBP* [109].

Substantial variation in central sBP was found across all categories of BP control, when defined according to guidelines (using office brachial BP and 24-hour ABPM). Risk stratification related to BP may be different from conventional approaches to management of AHT when central BP is considered in conjunction with both office brachial BP and out-of-office BP [69].

Parameters derived from office central arterial pressure waveforms were not useful for differentiating BP control in patients with AHT and highlight that central arterial BP cannot be assumed from the brachial BP measured in, or outside of, the office [111, 112]. The substantial overlap of central sBP across all categories of BP control assessed by 24-hour ABPM suggests that a combination of the information provided by measurement of central BP and out-of-office BP may be useful in clinical practice [69].

7. Treatment of MAHT

The main problem with MAHT is in its detection. Once diagnosed, it should be treated according to general principles. Lifestyle modifications are expected to help to the certain degree. With antihypertensives, care should be taken not to diminish BP too much in the hours when it is normal in the individual patient. Thus, antihypertensive drug and its dose should be tailored to prevent individual BP increases. Compelling indications are very important, indeed.

For many clinicians, *MAHT has unfortunately become a blind spot in antihypertensive therapy* [6]. As to the therapeutic approach, we should remember that WC-AHT has a benign prognosis and can only be overtreated; consequently, a conservative approach is probably justified. *Conversely, MAHT has a much more serious prognosis and can only be undertreated; it deserves, therefore, a thorough evaluation and a more aggressive therapeutic approach* [6].

At the current time, there is no treatment for MAHT that is based on trial data. Since nearly all patients with MAHT have elevated nocturnal BP (94% in the AASK Cohort), in the absence of trial data, there are several reasons why dosing medication at bedtime to lower nocturnal BP is a reasonable and safe approach. Studies have revealed that lower nocturnal BP does not increase risk of stroke and that bedtime dosing is also associated with lower awake BP. Lower nocturnal BP is linked to reduced proteinuria and there is some evidence from the Heart Outcomes Prevention Evaluation (HOPE) trial that it is also associated fewer CV events [20].

The HOPE study tested hypothesis that the addition of an ACE inhibitor (ramipril) will reduce major CV events compared to placebo in high-risk patients. In 75% of participants, ramipril was dosed at night, and therefore this study can be considered a nocturnal BP treatment trial. Twenty-four-hour BP was significantly reduced in the ramipril group compared with the placebo group (12/5 mmHg vs. 2/1 mmHg, P=0.03). A marked reduction in BP was observed in the ramipril group at night (16/7 mmHg, $P< 0.001$). Daytime BP reduction was not significant [20, 113].

Conclusion

Masked arterial hypertension deserves its name, because it can not be recorded in the office (where most often the diagnosis of arterial hypertension is made), without 24h ABPM. Moreover, it is still masked (unrecognized) for many colleagues.

Paradoxically, white-coat hypertension has been widely recognized and accepted, although it is far less dangerous in comparison to masked hypertension (which is not so recognized). Masked hypertension has been associated with hypertensive target organ damages, with significant comorbidity burden and with worse prognosis (as compared to normotensives and white-coat hypertensives).

References

[1] Pickering TG, White WB, Giles TD, Black HR, Izzo JL, Materson BJ, et al. When and how to use self (home) and ambulatory blood pressure monitoring. *J. Am. Soc. Hypertens.* 2010;4:56-61.

[2] O'Brien E. Is systolic blood pressure all that matters? No. *BMJ* 2009; 339: b2669

[3] Pogue V, Rahman M, Lipkowitz M, Toto R, Miller E, Faulkner M, et al.; African American Study of Kidney Disease and Hypertension Collaborative Research Group.

Disparate estimates of hypertension control from ambulatory and clinic blood pressure measurements in hypertensive kidney disease. *Hypertension* 2009;53:20-7.

[4] Messerli FH, Williams B, Ritz E. Essential hypertension. *Lancet* 2007; 370 (9587): 591-603.

[5] Pickering TG, Davidson K, Gerin W, Schwartz JE. Masked hypertension. *Hypertension* 2002; 40:795-6.

[6] Messerli FH, Cotiga D. Masked hypertension and white-coat hypertension:therapeutic navigation between scylla and charybdis. *J. Am. Coll. Cardiol.* 2005; 46:516-7.

[7] Cuspidi C, Negri F, Sala C, Mancia G. Masked hypertension and echocardiographic left ventricular hypertrophy: an updated overview. *Blood Press Monit.* 2012; 17: 8-13.

[8] Ishikawa J, Hoshide S, Eguchi K, Schwartz JE, Pickering TG, Shimada K, et al. Masked hypertension defined by ambulatory blood pressure monitoring is associated with an increased serum glucose level and urinary albumin-creatinine ratio. *J. Clin. Hypertens.* (Greenwich) 2010; 12: 578-87.

[9] Devereux RB, Pickering TG. Ambulatory blood pressure in assessing the cardiac impact and prognosis of hypertension. In: O'Brien E, O'Malley K, editors. *Blood pressure measurement*. Amsterdam: Elsevier; 1991. p 261-285.

[10] Kim SK, Bae JH, Nah DY, Lee DW, Hwang TY, Lee KS. Frequency and related factors of masked hypertension at a worksite in Korea. *J. Prev. Med. Public Health.* 2011; 44:131-9.

[11] Sega R, Trocino G, Lanzarotti A, Carugo S, Cesana G, Schiavina R, et al. Alterations of cardiac structure in patients with isolated office, ambulatory, or home hypertension: Data from the general population (Pressione Arteriose Monitorate E Loro Associazioni [PAMELA] Study). *Circulation* 2001;104:1385-92.

[12] Banegas JR, Segura J, Sobrino J, Rodríguez-Artalejo F, de la Sierra A, de la Cruz JJ, et al.; Spanish Society of Hypertension Ambulatory Blood Pressure Monitoring Registry Investigators. Effectiveness of blood pressure control outside the medical setting. *Hypertension* 2007;49:62-8.

[13] Belkić KL, Schnall PL, Landsbergis PA, Schwartz JE, Gerber LM, Baker D, et al. Hypertension at the workplace--an occult disease? The need for work site surveillance. *Adv. Psychosom. Med.* 2001;22:116-38.

[14] Wadei HM, Textor SC. Hypertension in the kidney transplant recipient. *Transplant. Rev.* (Orlando) 2010;24:105-20.

[15] Angeli F, Reboldi G, Verdecchia P. Masked hypertension: evaluation, prognosis and treatment. *Am. J. Hypertens.* 2010;23:941–8.

[16] Pierdomenico SD, Pannarale G, Rabbia F, Lapenna D, Licitra R, Zito M, et al. Prognostic relevance of masked hypertension in subjects with prehypertension. *Am. J. Hypertens.* 2008;21:879–83.

[17] Manios E, Michas F, Tsivgoulis G, Stamatelopoulos K, Tsagalis G, Koroboki E, et al. Impact of prehypertension on carotid artery intima-media thickening: actual or masked? *Atherosclerosis* 2011;214:215-9.

[18] Cohen DL, Townsend RR. Masked hypertension: an increasingly common but often unrecognized issue in hypertension management. *J. Clin. Hypertens.* (Greenwich) 2010; 12:522-3.

[19] Hanninen MRA, Niiranen TJ, Puukka PJ, Mattila AK, Jula AM. Determinants of masked hypertension in the general population: the Finn-Home study. *J. Hypertens.* 2011; 29:1980–8.
[20] Phillips RA. Controversies in blood pressure goal guidelines and masked hypertension. *Ann. N. Y. Acad. Sci.* 2012;1254:115-22.
[21] Baguet JP, Lévy P, Barone-Rochette G, Tamisier R, Pierre H, Peeters M, Mallion JM, Pépin JL. Masked hypertension in obstructive sleep apnea syndrome. *J. Hypertens.* 2008; 26:885-92.
[22] Ben-Dov IZ, Ben-Ishay D, Mekler J, Ben-Arie L, Bursztyn M. Increased prevalence of masked blood pressure elevations in treated diabetic subjects. *Arch. Intern. Med.* 2007; 167: 2139-42.
[23] Mann SJ, James GD, Wang RS, Pickering TG. Elevation of ambulatory systolic blood pressure in hypertensive smokers. A case-control study. *JAMA* 1991;265:2226-8.
[24] Pickering TG. The natural history of hypertension: prehypertension or masked hypertension? *J. Clin. Hypertens.* (Greenwich) 2007;9:807–10.
[25] Mallion JM, Clerson P, Bobrie G, Genes N, Vaisse B, Chatellier G. et al. Predictive factors for masked hypertension within a population of controlled hypertensives. *J. Hypertens.* 2006;24:2365–70.
[26] Trudel X, Brisson C, Larocque B, Milot A. Masked hypertension: different blood pressure measurement methodology and risk factors in a working population. *J. Hypertens.* 2009;27:1560–7.
[27] Minutolo R, Borrelli S, Chiodini P, Scigliano R, Bellizzi V, Cianciaruso B, et al. Effects of age on hypertensive status in patients with chronic kidney disease. *J. Hypertens.* 2007;25:2325–33.
[28] Pickering TG, Eguchi K, Kario K. Masked hypertension: a review. *Hypertens. Res.* 2007; 30:479–88.
[29] Eguchi K, Ishikawa J, Hoshide S, Pickering TG, Shimada K, Kario K. Masked hypertension in diabetes mellitus: a potential risk. *J. Clin. Hypertens.* (Greenwich) 2007; 9:601–7.
[30] Leitao CB, Canani LH, Kramer CK, Boza JC, Pinotti AF, Gross JL. Masked hypertension, urinary albumin excretion rate, and echocardiographic parameters in putatively normotensive type 2 diabetic patients. *Diabetes Care* 2007;30:1255–60.
[31] Charvat J, Chlumsky J, Szabo M, Zakovicova E, Zamrazil V. The association of masked hypertension in treated type 2 diabetic patients with carotid artery IMT. *Diabetes Res. Clin. Pract.* 2010;89:239-42.
[32] Uchida HA, Nakamura Y, Norii H, Kaihara M, Hanayama Y, Sada KE, et al. Insufficient control of morning home blood pressure in Japanese patients with hypertension associated with diabetes mellitus. *J. Diab. Investig.* 2010;1:266–72.
[33] Verberk WJ, Thien T, Kroon AA, Lenders JW, van Montfrans GA, Smit AJ, et al. Prevalence and persistence of masked hypertension in treated hypertensive patients. *Am. J. Hypertens.* 2007;20:1258-65.
[34] Kamoi K, Miyakoshi M, Soda S, Kaneko S, Nakagawa O. Usefulness of home blood pressure measurement in the morning in type 2 diabetic patients. *Diabetes Care* 2002; 25:2218–23.
[35] Mazze RS, Simonson GD, Robinson RL, endall DM, Idrogo MA, Adlis SA, et al. Characterizing blood pressure control in individuals with Type 2 diabetes: the

relationship between clinic and self-monitored blood pressure. *Diabet. Med.* 2003; 20:752–7.

[36] Kuriyama S, Otsuka Y, Iida R, Matsumoto K, Tokudome G, Hosoya T. Morning blood pressure predicts hypertensive organ damage in patients with renal diseases: effect of intensive antihypertensive therapy in patients with diabetic nephropathy. *Intern. Med.* 2005;44:1239–46.

[37] Rosenthal T, Alter A. Occupational stress and hypertension. *J. Am. Soc. Hypertens.* 2012; 6:2-22.

[38] Uzu T, Nakao K, Kume S, Araki H, Isshiki K, Araki S, et al. High sodium intake is associated with masked hypertension in Japanese patients with type 2 diabetes and treated hypertension. *Am. J. Hypertens.* 2012; 25:1170-4.

[39] Grassi G, Seravalle G, Trevano FQ, Dell'oro R, Bolla G, Cuspidi C, et al. Neurogenic abnormalities in masked hypertension. *Hypertension* 2007; 50:537–42.

[40] Papadopoulos DP, Perrea D, Thomopoulos C, Sanidas E, Daskalaki M, Papazachou U, et al. Masked hypertension and atherogenesis: the impact on adiponectin and resistin plasma levels. *J. Clin. Hypertens.* (Greenwich) 2009;11:61-5.

[41] Pérez-López FR, Larrad-Mur L, Kallen A, Chedraui P, Taylor HS. Gender differences in cardiovascular disease: hormonal and biochemical influences. *Reprod. Sci.* 2010; 17: 511-31.

[42] Lee SE, Kim HS. Human resistin in cardiovascular disease. *J. Smooth Muscle Res.* 2012; 48:27-35.

[43] Diagnosing hypertension -implications of the 2011 NICE guidance. *InnovAiT* 2012; 5: 204–9.

[44] Rodrigues TC, Canani LH, Viatroski RS, Hoffmann LH, Esteves JF, Gross JL. Masked hypertension, nocturnal blood pressure and retinopathy in normotensive patients with type 1 diabetes. *Diabetes Res. Clin. Pract.* 2010;87:240-5.

[45] Björklund K, Lind L, Zethelius B, Andrén B, Lithell H. Isolated ambulatory hypertension predicts cardiovascular morbidity in elderly men. *Circulation* 2003; 107:1297-302.

[46] Liu JE, Roman MJ, Pini R, Schwartz JE, Pickering TG, Devereux RB. Cardiac and arterial target organ damage in adults with elevated ambulatory and normal office blood pressure. *Ann. Intern. Med.* 1999; 131:564-72.

[47] Palatini P, Winnicki M, Santonastaso M, Mos L, Longo D, Zaetta V, et al. Prevalence and clinical significance of isolated ambulatory hypertension in young subjects screened for stage 1 hypertension. *Hypertension* 2004;44:170-4.

[48] Bobrie G, Chatellier G, Genes N, Clerson P, Vaur L, Vaisse B, et al. Cardiovascular prognosis of "masked hypertension" detected by blood pressure self-measurement in elderly treated hypertensive patients. *JAMA* 2004;291:1342-9.

[49] White WB, Maraka S. Is it possible to manage hypertension and evaluate therapy without ambulatory blood pressure monitoring? *Curr. Hypertens. Rep.* 2012;14: 366-73.

[50] O'Brien E. Twenty-four-hour ambulatory blood pressure measurement in clinical practice and research: a critical review of a technique in need of implementation. *J. Intern. Med.* 2011;269:478-95.

[51] Mancia G, Bombelli M, Facchetti R, Madotto F, Quarti-Trevano F, Polo Friz H, et al. Long-term risk of sustained hypertension in white-coat or masked hypertension. *Hypertension* 2009;54:226–32.
[52] Hare J, Sharman J, Thomas S, Leano T, Marwick T. Masked Hypertension is Common in Patients with a Hypertensive Response to Exercise and may Help to Explain Increased Cardiovascular Risk in this Population. *Heart, Lung and Circulation* 2008; 17,Suppl 3,S47.
[53] Delsart P, Philippe Marboeuf P, Delhaye C, Lablanche JM, Beregi JP, Mounier-Vehier C. Should we screen masked hypertension in patients with vascular disease? *Arch. Cardiovasc. Dis. Suppl.* 2010;2:75-9.
[54] Bangash F, Agarwal R. Masked hypertension and white-coat hypertension in chronic kidney disease: a meta-analysis. *Clin. J. Am. Soc. Nephrol.* 2009;4:656-64.
[55] Haydar AA, Covic A, Jayawardene S, Agharazii M, Smith E, Gordon I, et al. Insights from ambulatory blood pressure monitoring: diagnosis of hypertension and diurnal blood pressure in renal transplant recipients. *Transplantation* 2004;77:849-53.
[56] Kupferman JC, Singh A, Pavlakis SG. Lacunar stroke and masked hypertension in an adolescent male. *Pediatr. Neurol.* 2007; 36:125-7.
[57] Stabouli S, Kotsis V, Toumanidis S, Papamichael C, Constantopoulos A, Akopoulos N. White-coat and masked hypertension in children: association with target-organ damage. *Pediatr. Nephrol.*2005;20:1151-5.
[58] Wing LM, Brown MA, Beilin LJ, Ryan P, Reid CM. "Reverse white-coat hypertension" in older hypertensives *J. Hypertens.* 2002;20:639-44.
[59] Mancia G. Reversed white-coat hypertension definition, mechanisms and prognostic implications (editorial comment) *J. Hypertens.* 2002; 20: 579-81.
[60] O'Brien E. Unmasking hypertension. Hypertension 2005;45:481–2.
[61] Fagard RH, Cornelissen VA. Incidence of cardiovascular events in white-coat, masked and sustained hypertension versus true normotension: a meta-analysis. *J. Hypertens.* 2007; 25:2193–8.
[62] Ohkubo T, Kikuya M, Metoki H, Asayama K, Obara T, Hashimoto J, et al. Prognosis of ''masked'' hypertension and ''white-coat'' hypertension detected by 24-h ambulatory blood pressure monitoring 10-year follow-up from the Ohasama study. *J. Am. Coll. Cardiol.* 2005;46:508–15.
[63] Hansen TW, Kikuya M, Thijs L, Björklund-Bodegård K, Kuznetsova T, Ohkubo T, et al. Prognostic superiority of daytime ambulatory over conventional blood pressure in four populations: a meta-analysis of 7,030 individuals. *J. Hypertens.* 2007;25:1554–64.
[64] Lurbe E, Torro I, Alvarez V, Nawrot T, Paya R, Redon J, et al. Prevalence, persistence, and clinical significance of masked hypertension in youth. *Hypertension*2005;45:493-8.
[65] Ostrow V, Wu S, Aguilar A, Bonner R Jr, Suarez E, De Luca F. Association between oxidative stress and masked hypertension in a multi-ethnic population of obese children and adolescents. *J. Pediatr.* 2011; 158:628-633.e1.
[66] Wrobel MJ, Figge JJ, Izzo JL Jr. Hypertension in diverse populations: a New York State Medicaid clinical guidance document. *J. Am. Soc. Hypertens.* 2011;5:208-29.
[67] Rothwell PM. Limitations of the usual blood-pressure hypothesis and importance of variability, instability, and episodic hypertension. *Lancet* 2010;375(9718):938-48.

[68] Matsui Y, Eguchi K, Ishikawa J, Hoshide S, Shimada K, Kario K. Subclinical arterial damage in untreated masked hypertensive subjects detected by home blood pressure measurement. *Am. J. Hypertens.* 2007; 20:385–91.

[69] Schultz MG, Gilroy D, Wright L, Bishop WL, Abhayaratna WP, Stowasser M, et al. Out-of-office and central blood pressure for risk stratification: a cross-sectional study in patients treated for hypertension. *Eur. J. Clin. Invest.* 2012;42:393-401.

[70] Mitsnefes M, Flynn J, Cohn S, Samuels J, Blydt-Hansen T, Saland J, et al; CKiD Study Group. Masked hypertension associates with left ventricular hypertrophy in children with CKD. *J. Am. Soc. Nephrol.* 2010; 21:137-44.

[71] Tomiyama M, Horio T, Yoshii M, Takiuchi S, Kamide K, Nakamura S, et al. Masked hypertension and target organ damage in treated hypertensive patients. *Am. J. Hypertens.* 2006;19:880-6.

[72] Bobrie G, Clerson P, Menard J, Postel-Vinay N, Chatellier G, Plouin PF. Masked hypertension: a systematic review. *J. Hypertens.* 2008; 26: 1715-25.

[73] Clement DL, De Buyzere ML, De Bacquer DA, de Leeuw PW, Duprez DA, Fagard RH, et al. Prognostic value of ambulatory blood-pressure recordings in patients with treated hypertension. *N. Engl. J. Med.* 2003; 348: 2407-15.

[74] Marchesi C, Maresca AM, Solbiati F, Franzetti I, Laurita E, Nicolini E, et al. Masked hypertension in type 2 diabetes mellitus. Relationship with left-ventricular structure and function. *Am. J. Hypertens.* 2007; 20: 1079-84.

[75] Koracevic GP. Are some "lone" atrial fibrillations caused by masked hypertension? *Am. J. Hypertens*. 2012;25:838.

[76] Rafey M. Beyond office sphygmomanometry: ways to better assess blood pressure. *Cleve Clin. J. Med.* 2009;76:657-62.

[77] Pierdomenico SD, Lapenna D, Bucci A, Di Tommaso R, Di Mascio R, Manente BM, et al. Cardiovascular outcome in treated hypertensive patients with responder, masked, false resistant, and true resistant hypertension. *Am. J. Hypertens.* 2005;18:1422-8.

[78] Hänninen MR, Niiranen TJ, Puukka PJ, Johansson J, Jula AM. Prognostic significance of masked and white-coat hypertension in the general population: the Finn-Home Study. *J. Hypertens.* 2012;30:705-12.

[79] Pierdomenico SD, Cuccurullo F. Prognostic value of white-coat and masked hypertension diagnosed by ambulatory monitoring in initially untreated subjects: an updated meta analysis. *Am. J. Hypertens.* 2011; 24:52–8.

[80] Hansen TW, Jeppesen J, Rasmussen S, Ibsen H, Torp-Pedersen C. Ambulatory blood pressure monitoring and risk of cardiovascular disease: a population based study. *Am. J. Hypertens.* 2006;19:243–50.

[81] Mancia G, Facchetti R, Bombelli M, Grassi G, Sega R. Long-term risk of mortality associated with selective and combined elevation in office, home, and ambulatory blood pressure. *Hypertension* 2006;47: 846-53.

[82] Thaker N. Hypertension in children. *Apollo Med.* 2011;8:248–60.

[83] Hermida RC, Ayala DE, Mojón A, Fernández JR. Sleep-time blood pressure and the prognostic value of isolated-office and masked hypertension. *Am. J. Hypertens.* 2012; 25:297-305.

[84] Eguchi K, Hoshide S, Ishikawa J, Ishikawa S, Pickering TG, Gerin W, et al. Cardiovascular prognosis of sustained and white-coat hypertension in patients with type 2 diabetes mellitus. *Blood Press Monit.* 2008;13:15–20.

[85] Wijkman M, Länne T, Engvall J, Lindström T, Ostgren CJ, Nystrom FH. Masked nocturnal hypertension--a novel marker of risk in type 2 diabetes. *Diabetologia* 2009; 52:1258-64.

[86] Eguchi K, Hoshide S, Ishikawa S, Shimada K, Kario K. Aggressive blood pressure-lowering therapy guided by home blood pressure monitoring improves target organ damage in hypertensive patients with type 2 diabetes/prediabetes. *J. Clin. Hypertens.* (Greenwich) 2012; 14:422-8.

[87] Daskalopoulou SS, Khan NA, Quinn RR, Ruzicka M, McKay DW, Hackam DG, et al; Canadian Hypertension Education Program. The 2012 Canadian hypertension education program recommendations for the management of hypertension: blood pressure measurement, diagnosis, assessment of risk, and therapy. *Can. J. Cardiol.* 2012; 28: 270-87.

[88] Perk J, De Backer G, Gohlke H, Graham I, Reiner Z, Verschuren WM, et al. European Guidelines on cardiovascular disease prevention in clinical practice (version 2012): The Fifth Joint Task Force of the European Society of Cardiology and Other Societies on Cardiovascular Disease Prevention in Clinical Practice (constituted by representatives of nine societies and by invited experts). *Atherosclerosis* 2012;223:1-68.

[89] Stergiou GS, Salgami EV, Tzamouranis DG, Roussias LG. Masked hypertension assessed by ambulatory blood pressure versus home blood pressure monitoring: is it the same phenomenon? *Am. J. Hypertens.* 2005; 18:772-8.

[90] O'Brien E, Waeber B, Parati G, Staessen J, Myers MG. Blood pressure measuring devices: Recommendations of the European Society of Hypertension. *BMJ* 2001; 322: 531–6.

[91] Pickering T. Recommendations for the use of home (self) and ambulatory blood pressure monitoring. American Society of Hypertension Ad Hoc Panel. *Am. J. Hypertens.* 1996; 9:1–11.

[92] Pickering TG, Hall JE, Appel LJ, Falkner BE, Graves J, Hill MN, et al. Recommendations for blood pressure measurement in humans and experimental animals: part 1: blood pressure measurement in humans: a statement for professionals from the Subcommittee of Professional and Public Education of the American Heart Association Council on High Blood Pressure Research. *Circulation* 2005;111:697–716.

[93] Williams B, Poulter NR, Brown MJ, Davis M, McInnes GT, Potter JF, et al. Guidelines for management of hypertension: report of the fourth working party of the British Hypertension Society, 2004-BHS IV. *J. Hum. Hypertens.* 2004;18:139–85.

[94] Mancia G, De Backer G, Dominiczak A, Cifkova R, Fagard R, Germano G, et al. Guidelines for the management of arterial hypertension: The Task Force for the Management of Arterial Hypertension of the European Society of Hypertension (ESH) and of the European Society of Cardiology (ESC). *Eur. Heart J.* 2007;28:1462–536.

[95] Imai Y, Otsuka K, Kawano Y, Shimada K, Hayashi H, Tochikubo O, et al. Japanese society of hypertension (JSH) guidelines for selfmonitoring of blood pressure at home. *Hypertens. Res.* 2003;26:771–82.

[96] World Health Organization-International Society of Hypertension Guidelines for the Management of Hypertension. Guidelines Subcommittee. *J. Hypertens.* 1999; 17: 151–83.

[97] Chobanian AV, Bakris GL, Black HR, Cushman WC, Green LA, Izzo JL Jr, et al. The Seventh Report of the Joint National Committee on Prevention, Detection, Evaluation, and Treatment of High Blood Pressure: the JNC 7 report. *JAMA* 2003;289:2560–72.

[98] Hänninen MR, Niiranen TJ, Puukka PJ, Jula AM. Comparison of home and ambulatory blood pressure measurement in the diagnosis of masked hypertension. *J. Hypertens.* 2010; 28:709-14.

[99] Sundberg S, Kohvakka A, Gordin A. Rapid reversal of circadian blood pressure rhythm in shift workers. *J. Hypertens.* 1988;6:393–6.

[100] Sternberg H, Rosenthal T, Shamiss A, Green M. Altered circadian rhythm of blood pressure in shift workers. *J. Hum. Hypertens.* 1995;9: 349–53.

[101] Ben-Dov IZ, Bursztyn M. Is siesta masking masked hypertension? *Hypertension* 2007; 49:e25.

[102] Kario K, White WB. Early morning hypertension: what does it contribute to overall cardiovascular risk assessment? *J. Am. Soc. Hypertens.* 2008;2:397–402.

[103] White WB. Cardiovascular risk and therapeutic intervention for the early morning surge in blood pressure and heart rate. *Blood Press Monit.* 2001;6:63–72.

[104] Wroe SJ, Sandercock P, Bamford J, Dennis M, Slattery J, Warlow C. Diurnal variation in incidence of stroke: Oxfordshire community stroke project. *BMJ* 1992;304:155–7.

[105] Gallerani M, Manfredini R, Ricci L, Cocurullo A, Goldoni C, Bigoni M, et al. Chronobiological aspects of acute cerebrovascular diseases. *Acta Neurol. Scand.* 1993; 87:482–7.

[106] Kario K, Pickering TG, Umeda Y, Hoshide S, Hoshide Y, Morinari M, et al. Morning surge in blood pressure as a predictor of silent and clinical cerebrovascular disease in elderly hypertensives: a prospective study. *Circulation* 2003;107:1401–6.

[107] Li Y, Thijs L, Hansen TW, Kikuya M, Boggia J, Richart T, et al. Prognostic value of the morning blood pressure surge in 5645 subjects from 8 populations. *Hypertension* 2010; 55:1040–8.

[108] Dolan E, Stanton A, Thijs L, Hinedi K, Atkins N, McClory S, et al. Superiority of ambulatory over clinic blood pressure measurement in predicting mortality: the Dublin outcome study. *Hypertension* 2005;46: 156–61.

[109] Ben-Dov IZ, Ben-Arie L, Mekler J, Bursztyn M. Reproducibility of white-coat and masked hypertension in ambulatory BP monitoring. *Int. J. Cardiol.* 2007;117:355-9.

[110] Schultz MG, Hare JL, Marwick TH, Stowasser M, Sharman JE. Masked hypertension is "unmasked" by low-intensity exercise blood pressure. *Blood Press* 2011;20:284-9.

[111] McEniery CM, Yasmin, McDonnell B, Munnery M, Wallace SM, Rowe CV et al. Central pressure: variability and impact of cardiovascular risk factors: the Anglo-cardiff collaborative trial II. *Hypertension* 2008; 51:1476–82.

[112] Sharman J, Stowasser M, Fassett R, Marwick T, Franklin S. Central blood pressure measurement may improve risk stratification. *J. Hum. Hypertens.* 2008;22:838–44.

[113] Svensson P, de Faire U, Sleight P, Yusuf S, Ostergren J. Comparative effects of ramipril on ambulatory and office blood pressures: a HOPE Substudy. *Hypertension* 2001; 38:E28-32.

In: Arterial Hypertension
Editors: Marten Vosler and Siemen Weber

ISBN: 978-1-62417-852-8
© 2013 Nova Science Publishers, Inc.

Chapter 3

Arterial Hypertension: From Etiology to Treatment Options

Jing-bin Huang, Jian Liang, Xin Deng[*]
Wen-sen Wu and Xiao-fang Zhao
Department of Cardiothoracic Surgery, Ruikang Hospital Affiliated to Guangxi, University of Chinese Medicine, Nanning , Guangxi Zhuang Autonomous Region, China

Abstract

Arterial hypertension is one of the most frequent chronic diseases in the industrialized nations of the West and represents a major risk factor for cardiovascular morbidity and mortality. We review the evidence on practice-based approaches to improving blood pressure control, from new styles of patient education to home blood pressure monitoring. The conventional antihypertensive therapies including renin–angiotensin–aldosterone system antagonists (converting enzyme inhibitors, receptor blockers, renin inhibitors, and mineralocorticoid receptor blockers), diuretics, β-blockers, and calcium channel blockers are variably successful in achieving the challenging target blood pressure values in hypertensive patients. Difficult to treat hypertension is still a commonly observed problem world-wide. A number of drugs are considered to be used as novel therapies for hypertension. Renalase supplementation, vasopeptidase inhibitors, endothelin antagonists, and especially aldosterone antagonists (aldosterone synthase inhibitors and novel selective mineralocorticoid receptor blockers) are considered an option in resistant hypertension. In addition, the aldosterone antagonists as well as (pro)renin receptor blockers or AT2 receptor agonists might attenuate end-organ damage. This array of medications has now been complemented by a number of new approaches of non-pharmacological strategies including vaccination, genomic interference, controlled breathing, baroreflex activation, and probably most successfully renal denervation techniques. It remains an exciting question which approach will confer the best blood pressure control and risk reduction in this tricky disease.

[*]Corresponding author : Xin Deng MD, 10 Huadong Road, 530011, Nanning , Guangxi Zhuang Autonomous Region, China, email:hjb010222@163.com.

1. Introduction

Hypertension is defined by a systolic blood pressure that is ≥140 mm Hg and a diastolic blood pressure that is ≥90 mm Hg [1]. The World Health Organization ranks coronary heart disease and cerebrovascular diseases as the world's leading causes of death [2].

Globally, according to the World Health Report 2002, about 62% of cerebrovascular disease and 49% of ischemic heart disease are attributable to suboptimal blood pressure (systolic >115 mm Hg), and hypertension is estimated to cause 7.1 million deaths, about 13% of the total [3, 4].

According to the results of Kearney et al. [5], more than 25% of the world adult population (approx. 1 billion) has hypertension, and it was estimated that in 2025, 29% (1.56 billion) of the adult population will be hypertensive.

In spite of the huge amount of research recently performed in this area, the pathogenesis of human hypertension remains elusive. Thus, hypertension has to be defined as "essential" for the majority of patients with high blood pressure.

Given the lack of animal models useful to investigate essential hypertension, we analyze and discuss both clinical and basic research studies indicating that essential hypertension should be considered as a potential multifactorial inflammatory disease. The pathophysiology of essential hypertension might result from interactions between genetic and environmental factors.

2. Etiology

Despite extensive study, the etiology of most cases of human hypertension continues to be heavily debated. A number of factors increase BP, including (1) obesity, (2) insulin resistance, (3) high alcohol intake, (4) high salt intake (in salt-sensitive patients), (5) aging and perhaps (6) sedentary lifestyle, (7) stress, (8) low potassium intake, and (9) low calcium intake. [6] Furthermore, many of these factors are additive, such as obesity and alcohol intake.

Blood pressure regulation is a complex process involving renal, vascular and central mechanisms. The regulation of blood pressure (BP) is complex and multiple genes likely interact to influence BP, modulated by environmental contexts such as diet, physical activity, psychosocial factors, and aging.

2.1. Genes of Human Hypertension

Combining a classical linkage analysis with newly developed gene technology, the responsible genes of several monogenic forms of human hypertension have been dissected, and up to 20 of the candidate genes for human essential hypertension have been reported (Table 1). [7].

Table 1. Candidate Genes of Human Essential Hypertension

Locus	**Gene**
1p36 .2	Atrial Natriuretic Peptide
Locus	**Gene**
1q32	Renin
1q42-q43	Angiotensinogen
3q2 1-q25	Angiotensin II type 1 receptor
4p16 .3	α -adducin
5q31	Glucocorticoid receptor
5q32-q34	β_2 -adrenoreceptor
7p15-p13	Glucokinase
7q36	eNOS
8q22	Lipoprotein phospholipase
8p12 -pl 1.2	β_3-adrenoreceptor
8q21	Aldosterone synthase
10q24-q26	α_3-adrenoreceptor
11p15.5	Tyrosin hydroxylase
12p13	G protein β_3 -subunit
16p13.ll	S A
16p13 -p12	Na channel β -subunit
17q23	Angiotensin converting enzyme
19p13.2	Insulin receptor
19p13.2-p13.1	Low density lipoprotein receptor
19q13.3	glycogen synthase
19q13.3	Prostaglandin I_2 synthase
19q	kallikrein

Obesity is a major risk factor for the development of hypertension. Hypertension in obesity is commonly complicated by dyslipidemia and type 2 diabetes mellitus and hence imposes a high cardiovascular disease risk. Furthermore, obesity is strongly associated with resistant hypertension. Activation of the sympathetic nervous system and the renin-angiotensin system, leading to renal sodium and water retention, links obesity with hypertension. There is also evidence for the release of factors by visceral adipose tissue promoting excessive aldosterone production, and a more central role of aldosterone in obesity hypertension is emerging. Three mechanisms appear to be especially important in mediating increased sodium reabsorption associated with weight gain: (1) increased renal sympathetic activity, (2) activation of the renin-angiotensin system, and (3) altered intrarenal physical forces. Another mechanism, hyperinsulinemia, has also been suggested to raise arterial pressure in obese subjects. [8].

When sodium salt is loaded, factors that inhibit Na+, K+-ATPase activity increase in the circulating blood and in some tissues.[9] As inhibitors of Na+,K+-ATPase activity were identified as digitalis glycosides, they are termed 'endogenous digitalis-like factors' (EDLFs).[10] EDLFs include ouabain, digoxin, marinobufagenin (MBG), marinobufotoxin (MBT), telocinobufagin, proscillaridin A, bufalin and others. In recent years, EDLF has emerged as a key player, at least locally in the brain, in the onset of sodium-induced hypertension.[11]Renin mRNA expression was higher in rats fed a high-salt diet compared with control rats with a normal diet.[12]Similarly, expression of ACE mRNA and angiotensin type-1 receptor mRNA was higher in deoxycorticosterone acetate–salt hypertensive rats,[13] and ICV injection of Ang II causes far greater rises in blood pressure in those rats than in control rats. So, in contrast to its effect on PRA, sodium loading increases the activity of the brain renin–angiotensin system. Levels of aldosterone in the hypothalamus increase with sodium loading in rats, [14]suggesting that sodium loading activates the brain RAAS. Both Ang II and aldosterone injected ICV cause centrally induced increases in blood pressure.

2.2. The Central Nervous System and Inflammation in Hypertension

The brain is essential for processing and integrating neurohumoral signals from the periphery to maintain pressure and fluid homeostasis. Several distinct nuclei in the forebrain, hypothalamus and brainstem contribute to regulation of blood pressure and perturbations of these central sites contribute to the etiology of hypertension [15-17]. For example, human and experimental animal models of hypertension exhibit autonomic dysfunction, elevated sympathetic nerve activity (SNA) and altered baroreceptor sensitivity [17]. These neurogenic mechanisms are influenced by humoral factors such as angiotensin II and mineralcorticoids and by environmental factors such as stress and high salt intake. There is, however, emerging evidence that inflammation, and in particular adaptive immunity, contributes to hypertension.

Hypertension stimulates the accumulation of inflammatory cells including macrophages and T lymphocytes in peripheral tissues important in blood pressure control, such as the kidney and vasculature. Angiotensin II modulates blood pressure via actions on the central nervous system (CNS) and the adaptive immune system. Recent work suggests that the central actions of angiotensin II via the circumventricular organs lead to activation of circulating T-cells and vascular inflammation.

The bi-directional communication between the central nervous system (CNS) and the immune system are well known [18]. The sympathetic nervous system (SNS) and hypothalamic pituitary axis (HPA) are two major pathways that modulate this communication. The SNS innervates both primary (thymus, bone marrow) and secondary (spleen, lymph nodes, Peyer's patches) lymphoid tissues while most immune cells express receptors for neurohormones (i.e. glucocorticoids and angiotensin II) and for catecholamines (i.e. norepinephrine) [19]. Depending on immune cell type and level of activation, factors released from the HPA and SNS can have immunosuppressive and immuno-enhancing effects. Immunosuppressive effects of glucocorticoids, the end product of HPA axis activation, are well documented [20]. On the other hand, norepinephrine released from sympathetic nerve terminals can both enhance and inhibit adaptive and innate immune cells. Thus, the SNS and HPA can regulate the magnitude of innate or adaptive immune response in multiple ways. In reciprocal, the immune system also regulates the CNS. Pro-inflammatory cytokines produced in the periphery can feedback to the brain, passing through the blood brain barrier at leaky points such as the organum vasculosum lamina terminalis (OVLT) or median eminence. Interestingly, these brain regions, referred to as circumventricular organs (CVOs), are also essential to blood pressure and fluid homeostasis. In addition, cytokines can be produced locally in the brain by glia and neurons and contribute to a neuroinflammatory response implicated in neurodegenerative diseases and more recently identified in hypertension [21-23]. As proposed by Paton and colleagues [24], increased circulating inflammatory cells and cytokines in the brain can impair central blood pressure regulation and promote hypertension..

The neurohumoral effects of the RAS significantly contribute to the central regulation of blood pressure. Components of the RAS, including renin, angiotensinogen and angiotensin type 1 (AT1a) receptors are present in various brain regions and cell types [27–29]. The importance of the RAS and locally derived angiotensin II in the brain is highlighted by numerous studies where brain manipulations, such as lesioning of specific regions [30] and over expression of various components of the RAS in the brain [31] produce long term changes in blood pressure. In addition to brain-derived angiotensin II, blood-borne angiotensin peptides can enter the brain and modulate blood pressure and fluid homeostasis. Circulating angiotensin II accesses the CNS via the CVOs, which are hypothalamic regions around the third and fourth ventricles that have a weak blood brain barrier and contain a high density of angiotensin type 1 (AT1a) receptors. These regions include the OVLT, the area postrema (AP) and subfornical organ (SFO), and are essential to the regulation of blood pressure and fluid balance. In particular, the anteroventral third ventricle (AV3V) region, which encompasses periventricular neural structures including the OVLT and portions of the preoptic nucleus, has been well documented to play a role in various forms of hypertension. The AV3V region receives input from the SFO and sends efferent projections to key cardiovascular regulatory brainstem sites such as the nucleus of the solitary tract (NTS) and rostral ventrolateral medulla (RVLM). Electrolytic lesions that disrupt the AV3V region have been shown to virtually abolish all of the central actions of angiotensin II including drinking behavior, sympathetic outflow, vasopressin release as well as preventing and/or reversing several forms of experimental hypertension. ressure and how the neuroimmune link contributes to the etiology of hypertension.

Angiotensin II not only has important central effects in regulation of blood pressure, but also contributes to key events in inflammation[32]. For example, AT1a receptor blockade or anti-inflammatory treatment can lower blood pressure and reverse renal and vascular accumulation of inflammatory cells [33]. Moreover, angiotensin II dependent hypertension increases production of pro-inflammatory cytokines within specific brain regions involved in blood pressure control [23]. In addition, Zhang *et al.*, recently reported that angiotensin II increases permeability of the blood brain barrier and cerebral microvasculature inflammation [28]. Interestingly, other forms of experimental hypertension also promote inflammation in the brainstem microvasculature [24].

The relationship between angiotensin II and increased sympathetic nerve activity in hypertension are well documented [34, 35]. The SNS, as discussed above, can also impact the adaptive immune response in several ways. For example, T cell rich organs such as the spleen and lymph nodes are highly innervated with sympathetic nerves [36, 37]. Most immune cells possess adrenergic receptors, and T and B cells almost exclusively express the β2 subtype [38]. During increased sympathetic activation, norepinephrine released from the sympathetic nerve terminal has been shown to both inhibit and stimulate T cell activation and proliferation [39].

T cell activation and vascular inflammation by angiotensin II may be dependent on increased sympathetic outflow and catecholamine release or other central signals that were blocked by AV3V ablation. Alternatively, increased T cell activation and vessel inflammation during angiotensin II maybe secondary to the rise in blood pressure, which can be blocked by AV3V ablation. These recent studies clearly show that the central actions of angiotensin II on the CVOs contributes to increased systemic activation of T cells and vascular inflammation [40].

3. Pathophysiology

3.1. Volume Overload

The inability to excrete sodium and water via the kidneys contributes to increased extracellular volume, increased cardiac output, and increased BP. It is obvious that over the long term, there must be a precise balance between the intake and excretion of water and electrolytes and that chronic hypertension cannot develop unless there is a shift of renal-pressure natriuresis to higher blood pressures. However, total peripheral vascular resistance often increases during hypertension, even when hypertension is initiated by sodium retention and volume expansion, and the elevated blood pressure has also been suggested to be caused by direct or indirect effects of these hormones to constrict the peripheral vasculature. When renal perfusion pressure was servo-controlled during vasopressin or norepinephrine hypertension, there was continued sodium retention, marked volume expansion, and an inability to maintain sodium and water balance. [41-44].

3.2. Sympathetic Nervous System Activity

The technical progress in evaluating sympathetic nervous activity in humanhas accumulated evidence that sympathetic activity is frequently activated in essential hypertension, particularly in young hypertensive subjects [45, 46]. The plasma concentration of norepinephrine (NE) was elevated in young hypertensive subjects when data from various studies were pooled. Esler and colleagues demonstrated that spillover of NE from sympathetic neuroeffector junctions was elevated in essential hypertension, particularly in young hypertensive subjects. The increased spillover was evident in the heart, kidney and subcortical region of the forebrain, which would explain the hemodynamic characteristics of early hypertension, namely increased heart rate, cardiac output and renal vascular resistance. Direct microneurographicrecording of the sympathetic nerve traffic from the peroneal or brachial nerve has documented an increase in the sympathetic nerve activities (MSNA) in borderline hypertensive subjects with a further progressive increase in moderate and more severe hypertensive groups [46].

The renal sympathetic nerves can promote antinatriuresis directly through renal tubular innervation and indirectly by neurally mediated increases in renin release and renal vascular resistance [47]. Increased sympathetic activity appears to raise blood pressure mainly though the renal sympathetic nerves, because renal denervation blunted the sodium retention and markedly attenuated the rise in blood pressure associated with dietary obesity in dogs. Increased renal sympathetic nerve activity causes a parallel shift of the pressure natriuresis relationship to higher renal perfusion pressures in dogs. Chronic renal sympathetic nerve stimulation and NE infusion into the renal artery produced sustained hypertension in dogs and rats [47]. In sinoaortic denervated rabbits NaCl feeding produced hypertension that prevented by prior renal denervation [48]. An increase in renal vascular resistance and a decrease in renal blood flow are the most consistent abnormalities in benign essential hypertension. In many patients with essential hypertension of recent onset, the increased renal vascular resistance represents a functional abnormality which is sympathetically mediated [49]. Taken together with other extensive evidence, there is little doubt that increased activity of the sympathetic nervous system could be the cause of essential hypertension sustained by a sympathetic effect and later permanent renal changes to elevate the set point level of the kidney-body fluid pressure regulating mechanism [50]. Another mechanism by which the sympathetic nervous system maycontribute to the long-term regulation of arterial pressure is a trophic effect on vascular smooth muscle which promotes increasing vascular resistance and response to vasoconstrictor stimuli. Recent clinical and pathological studies have documented that patients with essential hypertension more frequently have neurovascular compression (NVC) of the rostral ventrolateral medulla, which is the major center of the sympathetic nervous system regulating the cardiovascular system, than subjects with secondary hypertension or normotension. Surgical neurovascular decompression is accompanied with a reduction in blood pressure. Blood pressure was reported to begin to decrease gradually 48 h after surgical decompression in patients with refractory hypertension [51].

Evidence will also be provided that sympathetic activation is a peculiar feature of essential hypertension, particularly in its early stages, with secondary forms of high blood pressure not usually characterized by an increased central sympathetic outflow. Humoral, metabolic, reflex, and central mechanisms are likely to be the factors responsible for the adrenergic activation characterizing hypertension, which may also promote the development and progression of the cardiac and vascular alterations that lead to hypertension-related morbidity and mortality, independent of blood pressure values. This represents the rationale for considering sympathetic deactivation one of the major goals of antihypertensive treatment. [52].

3.3. Renin-Angiotensin-Aldosterone System

The pharmacological RAAS inhibition reduces BP and represents a key part of current approaches to cardiovascular (CV) risk reduction. The classical simplified RAAS image has recently turned to a complex network. The cascade starts with the renal release of the renin, which cleaves the liver-produced angiotensinogen to angiotensin I (Ang I). [53] Renin may also bind to its (pro)rennin receptor (P)RR, [54] that enhances its cleavage activity and activates its inactive precursor, prorenin. However, binding to (P)RR elicits angiotensin-independent effects, such as activation of promyelocytic zinc finger (PLZF), protein-phosphatidylinositol-3-kinase and eventually mitogen-activated protein kinases (MAPKs) resulting in enhanced proteosynthesis, proliferation, and decreased apoptosis. [55-57] Angiotensin I (Ang I; Ang 1–10) formed by renin activity is hydrolysed by the circulating and locally expressed angiotensinconverting enzyme (ACE) to the active angiotensin II (Ang II; Ang 1–8). Angiotensin-converting enzyme also inactivates bradykinin with its nitric oxide (NO)- and prostacyclin (PGI2) stimulating and vasodilative activity. Ang II formation may take place independently of ACE via the enzymatic activity of chymase, carboxypeptidase, cathepsin G, or tonin. [58] In fact, Ang I catabolism is even more complex. Neutral endopeptidase (NEP) can cleave Ang I to Ang 1–7, [59] which may be formed by an ACE homologue, ACE2, via Ang 1–9 or directly from Ang II as well. [60] While Ang (1–7) is degraded by ACE to Ang (1–5), Ang II is degraded to Ang III and IV by aminopeptidase A (AMPA) and M (AMPM), respectively. [61] The different cleavage products then elicit various receptor affinities. Angiotensin type 1 receptor (AT1R) mediates most of the Ang II effects, which might be partially opposed by type 2 receptor (AT2R). Angiotensin III (Ang 2–8) displays affinity to AT1R and AT2R as well. AT2R is also activated by Ang (1–9), while Ang (1–7) stimulates the Mas receptor [62] and possibly theAT2R. [63] Finally,Ang IV(Ang 3–8) activates the AT4R or insulin-regulated aminopeptidase. [64] The AT1R mediates, among others, vasoconstriction, inflammation, myocardial and vascular hypertrophy, and fibrosis. It is one of the triggers [along with adrenocorticotropic hormone (ACTH), antidiuretic hormone, catecholamines, endothelin, serotonin, or Mg2+ and K+ levels] of aldosterone release, which contributes to Na+ retention and cardiac, vascular, and glomerular remodelling. [65] The AT2R, inhibits MAPKs, activates NO/cGMP and phospholipase A2 pathways, mediating thus anti-proliferation, vasodilation, and anti-inflammation. [66-69] The pharmacological stimulation of AT2R with the recently discovered non-peptide agonist, compound 21, improved myocardial function in rats with myocardial infarction independently of BP effects [70] but along with anti-inflammatory action and NF-kB inhibition. [71] Mas may also partially antagonize the AT1R effects. It promotes Akt phosphorylation,[72] NO release,[73] vasodilation, and antiinflammation. [74] Mas stimulation with a synthetic peptide induced vasorelaxation, reduced BP in spontaneously hypertensive rats (SHR) and showed antiarrhythmic effects [75] suggesting some therapeutic potential. Finally, AT4R stimulation results in proinflammatory effects with possible negative impact. This complex puzzle of the 'novel RAAS' complicates our understanding of mechanisms participating in the effects of RAAS-interfering drugs, but it offers new and promising drug targets, as well; rendering the RAAS far from being fully exploited.

PRA mainly reflects the activity of renal renin, but there is renin not only in salivary glands [76] but also in the brain. [77] Expression of renal renin mRNA markedly increases with sodium depletion and captopril treatment, whereas brain renin mRNA decreases. [78] Brain rennin may differ from that produced elsewhere as the end product, Ang II in the CNS, causes sympathetic activation and increases blood pressure. [79] Activation of the brain RAAS may be an essential cause of hypertension. If RAAS blockers affect central sites, it makes sense that they are effective even in low-renin essential hypertensives. Blood pressure increases after ICV injection of hypertonic saline are accompanied by increased peripheral sympathetic tone. [80, 81] In particular, renal nerve activity markedly increases with ICV injection of hypertonic saline, [82] and renal arterial blood flow, as measured with radioactive microspheres, decreases. [83] (Figure 1).

3.4. Oxidative Stress

Reactive oxygen species (ROS) are generated by multiple cellular sources, including NADPH oxidase, mitochondria, xanthine oxidase, uncoupled endothelium-derived NO synthase, cycloxygenase, and lipoxygenase. [84] The dominant initial ROS species produced by these sources is superoxide (O2−). Superoxide is short-lived molecule that can subsequently undergo enzymatic dismutation to hydrogen peroxide.

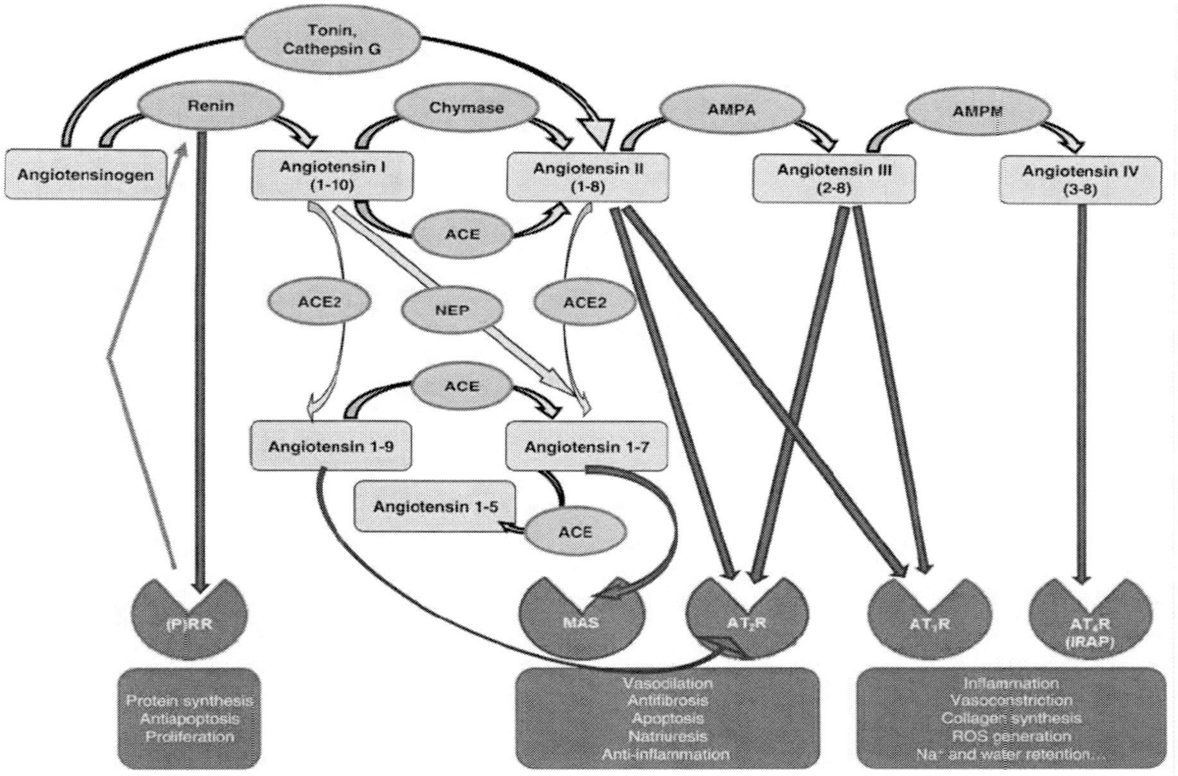

Figure 1. The interplay of recently discovered components of the renin–angiotensin–aldosterone system.

Superoxide can oxidize proteins and lipids, or react with endothelium-derived nitric oxide (NO) to create the reactive nitrogen species peroxynitrite Peroxynitrite and other reactive nitrogen species can subsequently oxidize proteins, lipids, and critical enzymatic cofactors that may further increase oxidative stress. [85, 86] The balance between superoxide production and consumption likely keeps the concentration of $O2-$ in the picomolar range and hydrogen peroxide in the nanomolar range. These homeostatic levels of reactive oxygen species appear to be important in normal cellular signaling[87, 88] and normal reactions to stressors. [89, 90] While multiple diverse factors likely contribute to the development of hypertension, the pathogenesis of this disease appears related, at least in part, to the development of a state of excessive oxidative stress. Local excessive superoxide production in the kidneys, CNS, and vasculature, along with inflammatory activation, are central findings in hypertension models. [91, 92] Animal studies demonstrate the development of hypertension with associated increases in oxidative stress and impaired vasodilation in rats exposed to a high-salt and oxidant containing diet. [93] Further, infusion of superoxide dismutase lowers oxidative stress and blood pressure in these animal models. Divergent animal models of hypertension, including spontaneous hypertension, [94] salt-sensitive hypertension, [95, 96] renovascular hypertension, [97, 98] and obesity-related hypertension[99] are all associated with excessive oxidative stress. These data suggest, regardless of etiology, excessive ROS is a common factor in the pathogenesis and morbidity of hypertension. The prominent role of excessive superoxide produced by NADPH oxidase under angiotensin II stimulation in the development of hypertension has recently been extensively reviewed.Mitochondria produce excessive ROS in the setting of spontaneous hypertension[100] as well as in hypertensive states characterized by salt-sensitivity and elevated endothelial-1 levels. [101, 102].

3.5. Arterial Stiffness

Arterial stiffness is a pathogenetic process that occurs naturally with aging, but is accentuated in disease states such as HTN, diabetes, and ESRD. Changes in the elastance properties of the walls of large arteries cause arterial stiffness. Healthy arteries are capable of accommodating the volume from each ventricular systolic ejection so that pressure waveforms reflected backwards from the peripheral circulation do not interfere with the forward transmission of another wave. However, stiffened, non-compliant arteries quickly transmit each ejected wave so that the timing of the reflected peripheral wave occurs while systole is still in progress. The ultimate consequence is increased systolic BP and pulse pressure, which contribute to LVH [103]. Arterial stiffness correlated with a diagnosis of HTN and pre-HD systolic BP, but not with average systolic BP.

4. Treatment Options

The goal of antihypertensive treatment is to reduce overall CVD risk and thus its morbidity and mortality rates. In any given patient, the decision to begin treatment is governed by the risk of CVD, which is determined by the magnitude of the BP elevation and the presence or absence of target organ disease and/or additional CVD risk factors. Recent consensus committees, including JNC VI and the World Health Organization–International Society of Hypertension (WHO-ISH) Guidelines Subcommittee, have modified traditional treatment recommendations in several important ways [104]: (1) Criteria for initiation of treatment now take into consideration total cardiovascular risk rather than BP alone, such that treatment is now recommended for persons whose BP is in the normal range but still bear a heavy burden of CVD risk factors or established CVD. (2) Systolic BP is recognized as an important target for treatment, particularly in older persons, because it is an even more important determinant of CVD risk than diastolic BP. (3) More aggressive BP goals are recommended for hypertensive patients with comorbid conditions such as diabetes mellitus or renal insufficiency. (4)

The importance of tailoring the choice of antihypertensive drug treatment to the patient's individual profile of concomitant CVD risk factors/comorbid conditions is emphasized. (5) The role of simultaneous reduction of multiple CVD risk factors in improving prognosis in hypertensive patients is stressed. (6)

Home and ambulatory BP measurement has been recommended because of its value in guiding therapy and enhancing adherence to treatment. (7) Greater reliance on evidence-based medicine (ie, results of randomized controlled trials with CVD outcomes) in making treatment decisions has been endorsed.

4.1. Lifestyle Modification

Lifestyle modifications are generally beneficial in reducing a variety of CVD risk factors (including high BP) and promoting good health and should therefore be used in all hypertensive patients, either as definitive treatment or as an adjunct to drug therapy. [105] Although sustained modifications in diet and lifestyle are difficult to achieve and have never been shown to reduce CVD morbidity or mortality rates in controlled trials, they may lower BP and obviate the need for drug treatment or reduce the dosages of antihypertensive drugs needed to control BP.

Therapy should be tailored to the individual characteristics of each patient, such as weight reduction and exercise for the overweight patient and moderate alcohol consumption for the heavy drinker.

A reasonable generalized approach for all patients includes (1) weight loss for the overweight patient; (2) regular physical activity; (3) moderation of alcohol consumption; (4) dietary modification to reduce sodium and fat and increase calcium, potassium, magnesium, vitamins, and fiber from food sources; and (5) cessation of smoking. Such an approach has been shown to produce significant sustained reductions in BP while reducing overall cardiovascular risk.

In well-motivated patients with stage 1 or 2 hypertension, modifying lifestyle effectively lowers BP and may be more important than the initial choice of antihypertensive drug. The same lifestyle modifications that are effective in treating hypertensive patients may be useful in the primary prevention of essential hypertension.

4.2. Weight Reduction

Weight loss is closely correlated with reduction in BP and appears to be the most effective of all nonpharmacological measures used to treat hypertension. Weight loss also enhances the efficacy of antihypertensive drugs. This effect is independent of dietary sodium restriction and is seen in both obese and nonobese hypertensive individuals. Weight reduction of as little as 10 lb reduces BP in a large proportion of overweight hypertensive persons and has a beneficial effect on associated coronary artery disease risk factors such as insulin resistance, diabetes, hyperlipidemia, and left ventricular hypertrophy, as well as the patient's self-image and sense of well-being. Weight reduction of at least 10 lb (with further increments depending on the initial response and the patient's baseline weight) through a combination of dietary caloric restriction and increased physical activity is recommended for all overweight hypertensive individuals. [104] These patients should avoid appetite suppressants, which contain sympathomimetics such as phenylpropanolamine that can elevate BP. The appetite suppressant drugs fenfluramine and phentermine have been withdrawn from the market because of cardiovascular toxicity, including serious mitral, aortic, and tricuspid regurgitant lesions and, rarely, pulmonary hypertension. Because sustained weight reduction is so difficult to achieve, more emphasis should be placed on prevention of weight gain, particularly in younger individuals with high normal BP and in families with a high prevalence of hypertension.

4.3. Increased Physical Activity

At least 30 minutes of moderately intense physical activity, such as brisk walking, swimming, bicycling, or yard work, at least 3 times per week (preferably once per day) can lower BP in both normotensive and hypertensive individuals. Studies suggest that such moderate activity may lower systolic BP by '4 to 8 mm Hg and is more effective than more strenuous forms of exercise such as running and jogging. [106] Additional benefits of regular physical activity include weight loss, enhanced sense of well-being, improved functional health status, and reduced risk of CVD and mortality from all causes. Accordingly, regular aerobic physical activity is recommended for all hypertensive individuals, including those with target organ damage. Patients with advanced or unstable CVD may require a medical evaluation before initiation of exercise or a medically supervised exercise program. Isometric exercise such as heavy weight lifting can have a pressor effect and should be avoided.

4.4. Moderation of Alcohol Intake

Alcohol consumption elevates BP both acutely and chronically. In cross-sectional and prospective studies involving all kinds of populations, the relationship between alcohol consumption, BP levels, and the prevalence of hypertension has been remarkably consistent. The relationship is linear, but some studies show a threshold effect of 2 to 3 drinks a day. The effect increases with age, is independent of the type of alcoholic beverage, and is additive but independent of the effects of obesity, oral contraceptives, and high salt intake. [107] Clinical studies show that BP falls 4 to 5 mm Hg in days or weeks with abstinence from alcohol. [108] However, moderate alcohol consumption (3 standard drinks a day) reduces overall CVD risk in the general population.[109] Whether this risk reduction also occurs in the hypertensive population needs to be studied further. Those having more than 2 standard alcohol drinks per day show an increase in both mortality rates and hypertension. It is estimated that in men, the contribution of alcohol to the prevalence of hypertension is 11%. [110] In nonobese heavy drinkers, systolic BP was '4 to 5 mm Hg higher than in nondrinkers. The mechanism by which alcohol raises BP is not known. Excessive alcohol intake also appears to cause resistance to antihypertensive therapy. For unrelated health reasons, alcohol consumption is not recommended for nondrinkers; for drinkers, intake should be limited to 1 oz of alcohol per day (2 oz of 100-proof whiskey, 8 oz of wine, or 24 oz of beer) in most men and half that amount in women and small men.

4.5. Dietary Modification

Two clinical trials, one with a comprehensive food plan that supplied the recommended dietary allowances of all major nutrients [111] and the other with a diet rich in fruits, vegetables, and low-fat dairy products and reduced in saturated and total fat, [112] produced reductions in BP comparable to or greater than those usually seen with monotherapy for stage 1 hypertension. The Dietary Approaches to Stop Hypertension (DASH) trial showed overall reductions in BP of 11.4/ 5.5 mm Hg in hypertensive persons on a diet rich in fruits, vegetables, and low-fat dairy products, compared with control subjects on a so-called "usual American diet," while dietary sodium intake and weight were held constant. The DASH "combination diet" also produced reductions in BP of 3.5/2.1 mm Hg in subjects without hypertension. Remarkably, subgroup analysis of the DASH trial indicated that the combination diet lowered BP effectively in all participating groups examined, independent of race, sex, age, BMI, level of education, income, physical activity, family history of hypertension, and geographic location of the study site. [112] The success of the DASH diet in lowering BP cannot be attributed solely to its micronutrient content (high in calcium, potassium, and magnesium) because the foods included in the DASH trial contain complex combinations of minerals, macronutrients, fiber, phytochemicals, vitamins, and other factors that alone or in combination could lower BP. [113].

4.6. Sodium Reduction

High sodium intake has generally been related to BP elevation, particularly in hypertensive individuals, and this effect appears to be augmented by concomitant low potassium intake. On the basis of these observations and the small but consistent BP-lowering effects observed in clinical trials of dietary sodium reduction in hypertensive subjects, particularly obese patients, older patients, blacks, and women, avoiding excessive sodium intake is recommended for all hypertensive individuals. Additional benefits of sodium reduction include reduced diuretic-induced hypokalemia and greater ease of BP control with diuretic therapy, protection from osteoporosis and fractures by reducing urinary calcium excretion, and favorable effects on left ventricular hypertrophy. A number of agencies have codified this recommendation as a reduction in daily consumption of sodium chloride to #6 g and of sodium to #2400 mg. [104, 114,115].

4.7. Potassium Repletion

Maintenance of adequate potassium intake (100 mmol/d), preferably from dietary sources, is recommended for hypertensive individuals and those with high normal BP. A diet rich in fruits and vegetables (DASH diet) is better than pills or other supplements as a source of potassium because these foods contain other nutrients, for example, calcium, magnesium, and vitamins, which may also have beneficial effects on BP. Moreover, it is clear that potassium supplements can be harmful and should be avoided or used only with extreme caution in patients with renal insufficiency, diabetics, and those receiving potassium-sparing diuretics, ACE inhibitors, or angiotensin II receptor blockers. [116].

4.8. Calcium Repletion

Although there is insufficient evidence to recommend high calcium intake for prevention or treatment of hypertension, calcium deficiency should be avoided. Inadequate calcium intake is common in populations at high risk of developing hypertension. Maintaining the recommended daily allowance for calcium, preferably from food sources, is beneficial for a variety of reasons, such as preventing osteoporosis. Furthermore, the DASH trial showed that a diet rich in low-fat dairy foods is associated with major reductions in BP in both normotensive and hypertensive persons. [111-113].

4.9. Smoking Avoidance/Cessation

Although cessation of smoking does not alter BP, it is important for the prevention of both CVD and non-CVD morbidity and mortality. All hypertensive patients who smoke should be counseled to stop, and nicotine replacement therapy should be considered. Measures to avoid or minimize weight gain after one stops smoking may be needed.

4.10. Pharmacological Treatment

Reducing BP by pharmacological means clearly reduces CVD morbidity and mortality rates. Benefits include protection from stroke, coronary events, heart failure, progression of renal disease, progression to more severe hypertension, and, most importantly, mortality from all causes. However, keeping patients on treatment and treating to a goal BP are difficult in practice, and ,25% of hypertensive patients in the United States are controlled (BP,140/90 mm Hg). [117] A major problem is the very high rate of discontinuance or change in medications by hypertensive patients: 50% to 70% of new treatments are changed or discontinued within the first 6 months in most practices. [105] Dealing with these barriers to adherence to prescribed therapy is the key to the successful treatment of hypertensive patients. Long-acting agents are preferable because adherence to therapy and consistency of BP control are superior when the drug is taken once a day. Low-dose, fixed-dose combination therapy can be used in place of monotherapy as initial treatment or as an alternative to adding a second agent of a different therapeutic class to unsuccessful monotherapy. Treatment should always include lifestyle modifications. For the minority of hypertensive patients without comorbid conditions, target organ damage, or concomitant CVD risk factors, JNC VI recommends starting drug therapy with a diuretic or b-blocker because (1) these are the only antihypertensive drugs shown to reduce CVD morbidity and mortality rates in randomized controlled trials, and (2) they are less costly than the newer classes of drugs. Despite the recent and substantial advances in the treatment of hypertension, the majority of patients still remains not optimally controlled; hence, the need for innovative strategies to lower blood pressure (BP). [118]. Novel approaches to hypertension treatment include: (i) drug-based strategies targeting traditional (e.g. the renin–angiotensin–aldosterone system, RAAS) or less-well studied (e.g. endothelin or renalase) neurohumoral pathways; (ii) unique approaches involving gene and vaccine therapies; and (iii) device-based therapies (baroreceptor sensitization or renal nerve ablation). [119, 200]. Angiotensin-converting enzyme inhibitors and AT1R blockers are in the centre of the current gold standard for cardioprotective therapies. Their beneficial effects are attributed to inhibition of the undesired AT1R stimulation and subsequent reduction in vascular tone, BP, aldosterone, vasopressin and catecholamines release, inhibition of inflammation, and attenuation of cell growth. There is a clear evidence for this approach given by clinical trials with ACE-Inhibitors. The later leave the AT2R unopposed for on-going Ang II stimulation and do not interfere with bradykinin catabolism, which is held responsible for the development of angioedema after ACE inhibition. Both ACE-Inhibitors and AT1R antagonists reduce the onset of new diabetes mellitus and some AT1R blockers, i.e. telmisartan or losartan with its metabolite EXP 3179, might offer even more metabolic protection as they have peroxisome proliferator-activated receptor-g activating properties.(Table 2)[201, 202].

Table 2. Number of selected compounds in development

Mechanism	Approved	In clinical/late preclinical phase	Note
Angiotensin-converting enzyme inhibitors	0	2	Includes imidapril approved in Japan; and NO-releasing enalapril
AT1 receptor blockers	3	3	Does not include compounds with dual action
Anti RAAS vaccines	0	2	
AT2 receptor agonists	0	1	
Vasopeptidase inhibitors	0	4	Including compounds with dual action
Aldosterone antagonists	1	3	
Calcium channel blockers	1	1	
β-Blockers	1	0	Includes nebivolol, NO-releasing blocker
Endothelin antagonists	0	3	Including compounds with dual action
Double combinations	7	5	
Triple combinations	3	0	

4.10.1. Renin as a Target

Renin, catalysing the rate limiting step in the RAAS cascade, represents a very attractive therapeutic target that was recently exploited by the introduction of the first-in-class selective rennin inhibitor, aliskiren. Renin inhibition is indeed associated with the attenuation of Ang I and Ang II levels and BP reduction. [203]Aliskiren reduced BP comparably to b-blockers1,[204]diuretics,[205]ACE–Inhibitors,[206] and AT1R blockers.[203] The possible benefit in renin inhibition might reside in the attenuation of plasma rennin activity which is increased by ACE inhibition or AT1R blockade. [207]On the other hand, the high renin levels after aliskiren treatment might escape from renin inhibition and aliskiren may not prevent binding of renin to the (P)RR. [208].

4.10.2. Prorenin Receptor

The binding of (pro)renin to the (P)RR6 up regulates the transforming growth factor-b1, plasminogen activator inhibitor-1, fibronectin, and collagen expression,[209] enhances protosynthesis, proliferation, and decreases apoptosis;7,8 beside the effects on (pro)renin catalytic efficiency itself. Because aliskiren does not inhibit the activation of the (P)RR by (pro)rennin, [210]the specific blockade of (P)RR could not only reduce the enzymatic activity but also prevent some Ang-independent effects of renin. A handling region peptide (HRP) inhibiting the binding of prorenin to (P)RR, completely abolished diabetic nephropathy even in AT1R knockout mice. It also reduced cardiac fibrosis in stroke-prone SHR and—as observed by an independent group—reduced cardiac hypertrophy and fibrosis in SHR fed high-salt diet [211].

4.10.3. Vasopeptidase Inhibitors

Beside ACE there are other metallopeptidases that convert vasoactive substances, such as ACE2, NEP, or endothelin-converting enzyme (ECE-1). Recent findings indicate a great potential for combined ACE/ECE inhibitors, [212] Neutral endopeptidase substrates belong to vasodilators as well as vasoconstrictors and the effect of NEP inhibition on BP is therefore very modest and variable. [213] The design of molecules inhibiting both ACE and NEP is very feasible. One of the most studied vasopeptidase inhibitors, omapatrilat, reduced BP in several models of experimental hypertension as well as in hypertensive subjects, similarly to sampatrilat. [215] The dual AT1R/NEP antagonism (angiotensin receptor and neprilysin inhibitors, ARNI) could show a more favourable tolerance profile.

4.10.4. Aldosterone Receptor Antagonists

Spironolactone and eplerenone are mineralocorticoid-receptor blocking agents (MRAs) used for to block the epithelial and non-epithelial actions of aldosterone. These compounds reduce BP, [216]diminish urine protein excretion, [217]and confer CV gain in heart failure apparently independently of volume alterations. [218] There is an evolving understanding of aldosterone as a downstream effector for some BP-independent Ang II-mediated unfavourable effects.[219] The BP reduction after spironolactone is conferred similarly in hypertensives with and without primary aldosteronism, independently of ethnicity and urinary aldosterone excretion and it occurs within weeks and Therapeutic perspectives in hypertension 2743 persists indefinitely. Spironolactone might also reduce the apnoeahypopnea index in patients with resistant hypertension and sleep apnoea. [220].

4.10.5. Aldosterone Synthase Inhibitors

Another approach to antagonise aldosterone is to inhibit its formation and hence prevent the reactive increase in aldosterone levels and their MR-independent effects. Several aldosterone synthase (CYP11B2) inhibitors are being developed. Fadrozole, an aromatase inhibitor or its dextroenantiomer (FAD286) has been shown to inhibit aldosterone synthase and to reduce mortality, cardiac hypertrophy, albuminuria, cell infiltration, and matrix deposition in the kidney in double transgenic rennin rats (dTGR), yet without a profound effect on BP. [221]Similarly in Dahl salt-sensitive rats: intracerebroventriculary applied spironolactone fully eliminated the salt-diet-related increase in BP; whereas, FAD286 only prevented 30 mmHg of the 50 mmHg increase.[222] FAD286 and MRAs comparably reduced hypertrophy and interstitial fibrosis of the kidney and heart induced by Ang II and a high-salt intake.[223].

4.10.6. Endothelin System

From the endothelin (ET-1, ET-2, and ET-3) polypeptide family is ET-1, the most clinically pertinent isoform, which was identified in 1988 as a potent vasoconstrictor. It plays a prominent role in fibrogenesis, inflammation, oxidative stress, atherosclerosis, salt and water homeostasis, and pulmonary artery hypertension as well.[224] Endothelin receptor A (ETA) and B (ETB) antagonists have been studied in resistant hypertension with darusentan (ETA/ETB antagonist) being the one most extensively evaluated.[225] In patients with resistant hypertension, darusentan met the end-points for systolic and diastolic BP in the DAR-311 (DORADO) trial, and it produced a greater reduction in mean 24-h systolic and diastolic BP than either placebo or the central a2-agonist, guanfacine, in the DAR-312 (DORADO-AC) trial.[225] Endothelin antagonists have only been approved for use in pulmonary artery hypertension and their future for the treatment of hypertension is not particularly bright. The most pronounced sticking points with endothelin antagonists include prominent side-effect profile (salt and water retention and peripheral oedema), [226] high teratogenicity potential (FDA Pregnancy Category X), and propensity to dose-dependent transaminitis. [226].

4.10.7. Renalase System

Recently, in an extensive search for vasoactive kidney-related proteins, a novel catecholamine peptidase, renalase, was discovered. [227] Its basal plasmatic activity is very low, but it can be increased by catecholamines, which it in turn metabolizes. Kidneys are probably the major source of circulating renalase as in subnephrectomized rats or in patients with end-stage renal failure the renalase production in the heart, muscle, or liver could not compensate the deficit of kidney-produced renalase. [228]Renalase down-regulation or knock-out is associated with increased catecholamine levels, BP and higher susceptibility to ischaemic myocardial damage, [229]which are prevented by supplementation with recombinant renalase. Because one renalase polymorphism was associated with essential hypertension [230] and increased CV risk in patients with coronary heart disease. Regardless of the therapeutic potential and safety of renalase administration, its discovery might have provided a novel important pathophysiological link between the kidney, sympathetic tone, and BP.

4.11. Triple Therapies

A considerable legacy, dating to the 1950s, exists for fixed-dose combination therapies. The rationale to this approach has remained constant since that time: combinations reduce BP because each drug blocks different effector pathways or the second drug checks counter-regulatory system activity triggered by the other.[231] In fact most of the hypertensive patients require at least two drugs to achieve the target BP values,[232] as recommended for mild-severe hypertension (≥grade 2) by the current guidelines. The addition of the diuretic hydrochlorothiazide to AT1R antagonists can markedly enhanced BP reduction and the combination of AT1R antagonist with Ca2+ channel blocker amlodipine was more effective compared with either drug alone. In addition to superior BP control, the addition ofAT1R antagonist might reduce the risk of peripheral oedema caused by amlodipine therapy [233] or hypokalaemia evoked by diuretic administration. Since 2000, 10 new fixed-dose combinations were approved including AT1R antagonist (or ACE-Inhibitor or renin inhibitor) + hydrochlorothiazide (and/or amlodipine); AT1R antagonist + renin inhibitor; ACE-Inhibitor + b-blocker; and amlodipine + statin [234] and their efficacy and safety has been established. However, the two-drug fixed-dose combination era is now rapidly morphing to three drug combinations. The investigational triple therapies are composed of a RAAS inhibitor, amlodipine, and hydrochlorothiazide.[235] In hypertensive patients with a mean sitting diastolic BP of .100 mmHg such triple-therapy (valsartan + amlodipine + hydrochlorothiazide) lowered BP by 40/25 mmHg which was significantly more compared with the any two-drug combination (Figure 3). [236]Although, unsurprisingly, the triple combinations provided more profound BP reduction and higher BP control rate without compromising the tolerability or safety, the question remains whether combination therapy should be administered in fixed-dose combinations or not. The advantages of single pill regimens are (i) more simple administration, (ii) more rapid achievement of BP goal than by gradual titration; (iii) existing simple and rapid full dose up-titration schemes; (iv) better patient adherence to therapy; (v) potential for fewer nonresponders to a three-drug choice. On the other hand, their disadvantages include (i) higher risk of dose-independent adverse reactions, (ii) loss of dose flexibility, with possibly inappropriate dosing, [236] and (iii) the inability to introduce a chronotherapeutic approach. Hence, individually tailored therapy is traded for reduced costs and simplification. More studies on novel combinations including aliskiren as RAAS inhibitor or chlorthalidone as diuretic are on the way and the recommendations on triple therapy should become more specific. After more evidence is provided, patients that will mostly benefit from single-pill regimens can be identified, while in others the therapy may still be individually adjusted.

4.12. Gene-based Therapies

The pharmacological approaches, including the investigational ones, represent ‘only’ a possible treatment option for hypertension. With complete genome sequenced and other advances in genetics and genetic manipulations there is a search for longerlasting solution for hypertension meaning better patient compliance, 24-h BP control and possible cost reduction. Some data are encouraging. Overexpression of ACE2 and AT2R delivered in viral vectors reduced cardiac remodeling [237] and potentiated BP control by losartan in rats with chronic

Ang II infusion. Adenoviral transfer of endothelial NO-synthase and kallikrein genes improved endothelial dysfunction [238] and cardiac remodeling in SHR. Even more promising results were reported with suppression of vasoconstrictor expression by the use of cDNA antisense. In SHR, virally delivered antisense cDNA against ACE and AT1R [239] reduced respective gene expression and attenuated BP. On the other hand a delivery of kallikrein gene in pure plasmid cDNA p.o. reduced BP in SHR but only for 3–5 days. [240] Alternative delivery systems include the use of antisense oligodeoxynucleotides and small interfering (si)RNA. Small interfering RNA against the prepro-thyrotropin-releasing hormone in obesity-induced hypertensive rats reduced BP for at least 24 days. [241] Although being exciting, until more safe and reliable methods of nucleic acid transfer are established, gene-based therapies are unlikely to offer substantial advantage over pharmacological therapies and will rather provide a valuable experimental tool.

4.13. Vaccine-Based Strategies

An immunological approach might offer similar advantages to those expected from gene-based strategies. Recently, two antihypertensive vaccines were developed: PMD3117 against Ang I and Cyt006 against Ang II. Despite some excitement the results were rather disappointing. Although Cyt006 reduced BP in SHR, [242] it achieved inferior BP reduction (9/4 mmHg) [243] compared with conventional antihypertensives. The vaccination approach seems feasible and might lead to more effective vaccines or their preventive employment against CV diseases.

4.14. Novel Device-Based Approaches

4.14.1. Controlled Breathing

Yoga, meditation, and music decrease sympathetic nervous system activity, sensitize arterial and cardiopulmonary baroreceptors and in so doing reduce BP lability and elevated resting BP values. Similarly, slow breathing (,10b.p.m.), especially with a component of prolonged exhalation, reduced sympathetic nerve traffic while increasing parasympathetic activity and lowered BP.[244] Slow breathing can be achieved by systems that coach patients to coordinate their breathing with music, which gradually entrains the respiratory rate downward. The systems require two 15-min sessions daily, endeavouring to achieve at least 45 min of slow breathing time per week. A stored record of the session can be used to assess the patients' adherence. While there are no known contraindications and no reported adverse events, this technique requires a fair amount of discipline and some patients may view pill taking for BP control to be less time-consuming. Moreover, poor hearing (frequent in the elderly) complicates use of this device and a persisting BP-lowering effect seems unlikely. Therefore, the device might find its use as an adjunctive antihypertensive treatment complementing other pharmacological and/or non-pharmacological interventions. [245] All in all, the published information on this device is sparse and the reported studies lack the comparison to techniques such as meditative relaxation to estimate the contribution of a placebo effect to the BP response.

4.14.2 Renal Sympathetic Denervation

Renal nerve ablation has been advanced as a means to interrupting the varied mechanistic pathways by which the kidney affects BP. [246] Recently, a percutaneous, catheter-based radiofrequency ablation for renal sympathetic denervation has been developed. This procedure has been evaluated in a cohort study of 45-treated patients with treatment resistant hypertension. The safety and effectiveness of catheter-based renal denervation for reduction of BP was assessed in 106 patients with resistant hypertension. [247] This procedure hold considerable promise for the patients with resistant hypertension but the specific baseline predictors of success and head-to-head comparisons with other drugs, such as aldosterone antagonists, are yet to be determined. [248].

4.14.3. Baroreceptor Activation

The concept of treating hypertension by prolonged electrical activation of the carotid baroreflex has existed since the mid-1960s when clinical studies were initiated in patients with severe hypertension refractory to medication. [249] Recently, the development of the three-component Rheosw Hypertension System has resurrected this approach. [250] In the Rheosw DEBuT-HT trial on 45 patients, 72% of 18 patients (baseline BP of 193+36/111+20 mmHg and heart rate of 74+ 13 b.p.m.) treated for 58+6 months achieved at least a 30-mmHg drop in systolic BP at 4 years (253+9 mmHg) and the average number of antihypertensive medications used fell from 5.0 to 3.4. [251, 252].

Conclusion

Difficult to treat hypertension is a commonly observed problem globally. Available, conventional therapies have been the mainstay of therapy for hypertension but still have been variably successful in bringing BP to goal. A number of other drug classes have been used as complementary therapies for BP reduction including central a2-receptor agonists, peripheral a1-receptor antagonists, and direct vasodilators. This array of medications has now been complemented by a number of new approaches of a medication, immunologic, and device nature.

Many of them are being tested and the basis for their use refined. In addition, therapeutic regimens are being fine-tuned and several novel fixed-dose combinations were recently established. However, therapies such as aldosterone synthase inhibition, endothelin receptor antagonism, and gene and vaccine based-strategies have evolved more slowly than expected and point to the difficulty in bringing a new therapy for hypertension to market.

Acknowledgments

This study was supported by the Ruikang Hospital Natural Science Foundation (code:ZKZ201001).

References

[1] Mancia G, de Backer G, Dominiczak A, et al. 2007 Guidelines for the management of arterial hypertension: the Task Force for the Management of Arterial Hypertension of the European Society of Hypertension (ESH) and of the European Society of Cardiology (ESC). *J Hypertens* 2007; 25: 1105–1187.
[2] World Health Organization: Fact Sheet: The Top Ten Causes Of Death. Fact sheet No. 310. Geneva, WHO, 2008.
[3] World Health Organization: The World Health Report 2002: Reducing Risks, Promoting Healthy Life. Geneva, WHO, 2002.
[4] Murray CJL, Lopez AD: Global mortality, disability, and the contribution of risk factors: Global Burden of Disease Study. *Lancet* 1997; 349: 1436–1442.
[5] Kearney PM, Whelton M, Reynolds K, et al. Global burden of hypertension: analysis of worldwide data. *Lancet* 2005; 365: 217–223.
[6] Oscar A. Carretero, Suzanne Oparil. Essential Hypertension : Part I: Definition and Etiology. *Circulation.* 2000;101:329-335.
[7] Symposium on The Etiology of Hypertension:Summerizing Studies in 20th Century. *Internal Medicine* 2001; 40:144-147.
[8] John EH.The Kidney, Hypertension, and Obesity. *Hypertension.*2003;41:625-633
[9] Hakuo T, Masamichi Y, Yutaka K, et al. The central mechanism underlying hypertension: a review of the roles of sodium ions, epithelial sodium channels, the renin–angiotensin–aldosterone system, oxidative stress and endogenous digitalis in the brain. *Hypertension Research* 2011; 34:1147–1160.
[10] Hamlyn JM, Levinson PD, Ringel R, et al. Relationships among endogenous digitalis-like factors in essential hypertension. *Fed Proc* 1985; 44: 2782–2788.
[11] Graves SW, Williams GH. Endogenous digitalis-like natriuretic factors. *Annu Rev Med* 1987; 38: 433–444.
[12] Tymiak AA, Norman JA, Bolgar M, et al. Physicochemical characterization of a ouabain isomer isolated from bovine hypothalamus. *Proc Natl Acad Sci USA* 1993; 90: 8189–8193.
[13] Nishimura M, Ohtsuka K, Takahashi H, et al. Role of FMRFamide-activated brain sodium channel in salt-sensitive hypertension. *Hypertension* 2000; 35: 443–450.
[14] Huang BS, Cheung WJ, Wang H, et al. Activation of brain renin-angiotensin-aldosterone system by central sodium in Wistar rats. *Am J Physiol* 2006; 291: H1109–H1117.
[15] Paul JM, Heinrich L, Antony V, et al. The Central Nervous System and Inflammation in Hypertension. *Curr Opin Pharmacol.* 2011; 11: 156–161.
[16] Paton JF, Raizada MK. Neurogenic hypertension. *Exp Physiol.* 2010; 95:569–571.
[17] Shi P, Diez-Freire C, Jun JY, et al. Brain microglial cytokines in neurogenic hypertension. *Hypertension.* 2010; 56:297–303.
[18] Elenkov IJ, Wilder RL, Chrousos GP, et al. The sympathetic nerve--an integrative interface between two supersystems: the brain and the immune system. *Pharmacol Rev.* 2000; 52:595–638.
[19] Nance DM, Sanders VM. Autonomic innervation and regulation of the immune system (1987–2007). *Brain Behav Immun.* 2007; 21:736–745.

[20] Webster JI, Tonelli L, Sternberg EM. Neuroendocrine regulation of immunity. *Annu Rev Immunol.*2002; 20:125–163.

[21] Agostinho P, Cunha RA, Oliveira C. Neuroinflammation, oxidative stress and the pathogenesis of Alzheimer's disease. *Curr Pharm Des*. 2010; 16:2766–2778.

[22] Paton JF, Waki H, Abdala AP, et al. Vascular-brain signaling in hypertension: role of angiotensin II and nitric oxide. *Curr Hypertens Rep*. 2007; 9:242–247.

[23] Shi P, Raizada MK, Sumners C. Brain cytokines as neuromodulators in cardiovascular control. *Clin Exp Pharmacol Physiol.* 2010; 37:e52–e57.

[24] Paton JF, Waki H. Is neurogenic hypertension related to vascular inflamma tion of the brainstem? *Neurosci Biobehav Rev*. 2009; 33:89–94.

[25] Benigni A, Cassis P, Remuzzi G. Angiotensin II revisited: new roles in inflammation, immunology and aging. *EMBO Mol Med*. 2010; 2:247–257.

[26] Rodriguez-Iturbe B, Quiroz Y, Nava M, et al. Reduction of renal immune cell infiltration results in blood pressure control in genetically hypertensive rats. *Am J Physiol Renal Physiol*. 2002; 282:F191–F201.

[27] McKinley MJ, Albiston AL, Allen AM, et al. The brain renin-angiotensin system: location and physiological roles. *Int J Biochem Cell Biol*. 2003; 35:901–918.

[28] Guzik TJ, Hoch NE, Brown KA, et al. Role of the T cell in the genesis of angiotensin II induced hypertension and vascular dysfunction. *J Exp Med*. 2007; 204:2449–2460.

[29] Hoch NE, Guzik TJ, Chen W, et al. Regulation of T-cell function by endogenously produced angiotensin II. *Am J Physiol Regul Integr Comp Physiol.* 2009; 296:R208–R216.

[30] Shan Z, Shi P, Cuadra AE, et al. Involvement of the brain (pro)renin receptor in cardiovascular homeostasis. *Circ Res*. 2010; 107:934–938.

[31] Hendel MD, Collister JP. Contribution of the subfornical organ to angiotensin II-induced hypertension. *Am J Physiol Heart Circ Physiol*. 2005; 288:H680–H685.

[32] Marvar PJ, Thabet SR, Guzik TJ, et al. Central and peripheral mechanisms of T-lymphocyte activation and vascular inflammation produced by angiotensin II-induced hypertension. *Circ Res*. 2010; 107:263–270.

[33] Harrison DG, Vinh A, Lob H, et al. Role of the adaptive immune system in hypertension. *Curr Opin Pharmacol*. 2010; 10:203–207.

[34] Crowley SD, Song YS, Lin EE, et al. Lymphocyte responses exacerbate angiotensin II-dependent hypertension. *Am J Physiol Regul Integr Comp Physiol.* 2010; 298:R1089–R1097.

[35] De Miguel C, Das S, Lund H, et al. T lymphocytes mediate hypertension and kidney damage in Dahl salt-sensitive rats. *Am J Physiol Regul Integr Comp Physiol.* 2010; 298:R1136–R1142.

[36] Grobe JL, Dickson ME, Park S, et al. Cardiovascular consequences of genetic variation at -6/235 in human angiotensinogen using "humanized" gene-targeted mice. *Hypertension*. 2010; 56:981–987.

[37] Viel EC, Lemarie CA, Benkirane K, et al. Immune regulation and vascular inflammation in genetic hypertension. *Am J Physiol Heart Circ Physiol.* 2010; 298:H938–H944.

[38] Osborn JW, Fink GD. Region-specific changes in sympathetic nerve activity in angiotensin II-salt hypertension in the rat. *Exp Physiol*. 2010; 95:61–68.

[39] Malpas SC. Sympathetic nervous system overactivity and its role in the development of cardiovascular disease. *Physiol Rev*. 2010; 90:513–557.
[40] Kin NW, Sanders VM. CD86 stimulation on a B cell activates the phosphatidylinositol 3- kinase/Akt and phospholipase C gamma 2/protein kinase C alpha beta signaling pathways. *J Immunol.*2006; 176:6727–6735.
[41] Hall JE, Mizelle HL, Hildebrandt DA, Brands MW. Abnormal pressure natriuresis: a cause or a consequence of hypertension? *Hypertension*. 1990;15:547–559.
[42] John EH. The Kidney, Hypertension, and Obesity. *Hypertension*. 2003;41:625-633
[43] Hall JE, Guyton AC, Brands MW. Pressure-volume regulation in hypertension. *Kid Int.* 1996;49:S35–S41.
[44] Hall JE, Brands MW, Shek EW. Central role of the kidney and abnormal fluid volume control in hypertension. *J Hum Hypertens*. 1996;10: 633–639.
[45] Mark AL. The sympathetic nervous system in human hypertension: a potential long-term regulator of arterial pressure. *J Hypertens* 14 (suppl 5): S159-S165, 1996.
[46] Grassi G. Role of the sympathetic nervous system in human hypertension. J Hypertens 16: 1979-1987, 1998.
[47] DiBona GF, Kopp UC. Neural control of renal function. *Physiol Rev* 77: 75-197, 1997.
[48] Ryuzaki M, Suzuki H, Kumagai K, et al. Renal nerves contribute to salt induced hypertension in sinoaortic denervated uninephrectomized rabbits. *Am J Physiol* 262: R733-R737, 1992.
[49] Ruilope LM, Lahera V, Rodicio JL, et al. Are renal hemodynamics a key factor in the development and maintenance of arterial hypertension in humans? *Hypertension* 23: 3-9, 1994.
[50] Guyton AC. Hypertension: a neural disease? *Arch Neurol* 1988; 45: 178-179
[51] Geiner H, Naraghi R, Schobel HP, et al. Decrease of blood pressure by ventrolateral medullary decompression in essential hypertension. *Lancet* 352: 446-449, 1998.
[52] Shuichi T. The Sympathetic Nervous System in Essential Hypertension: *Pathophysiological Significance. Internal Medicine* 2001;40:151-153.
[53] Unger T. The role of the renin-angiotensin system in the development of cardiovascular disease. *Am J Cardiol* 2002;89:3A–9A.
[54] Nguyen G, Delarue F, Burckle′ C, et al. Pivotal role of the renin/prorenin receptor in angiotensin II production and cellular responses to renin. *J Clin Invest* 2002;109:1417–1427.
[55] Schefe JH, Menk M, Reinemund J, et al. A novel signal transduction cascade involving direct physical interaction of the renin/prorenin receptor with the transcription factor promyelocytic zinc finger protein. *Circ Res* 2006;99:1355–1366.
[56] Schefe JH, Unger T, Funke-Kaiser H. PLZF and the (pro)renin receptor. *J Mol Med* 2008;86:623–627.
[57] Funke-Kaiser H, Zollmann FS, Schefe JH, et al. Signal transduction of the (pro)renin receptor as a novel therapeutic target for preventing end-organ damage. *Hypertens Res* 2010;33:98–104.
[58] Johnston CI, Risvanis J. Preclinical pharmacology of angiotensin II receptor antagonists: update and outstanding issues. *Am J Hypertens* 1997;10:306S–310S.
[59] Welches WR, Brosnihan KB, Ferrario CM. A comparison of the properties and enzymatic activities of three angiotensin processing enzymes: angiotensin converting

enzyme, prolyl endopeptidase and neutral endopeptidase 24.11. *Life Sci* 1993;52:1461–1480.

[60] Donoghue M, Hsieh F, Baronas E, et al. A novel angiotensin-converting enzyme-related carboxypeptidase (ACE2) converts angiotensin I to angiotensin1–9. *Circ Res* 2000;87:E1–E9.

[61] Fyhrquist F, Saijonmaa O. Renin-angiotensin system revisited. *J Intern Med* 2008; 264:224–236.

[62] Santos RA, Simoes e Silva AC, Maric C, et al. Angiotensin-(1–7) is an endogenous ligand for the Gprotein-coupled receptor Mas. *Proc Natl Acad Sci U S A* 2003;100:8258–8263.

[63] Lara Lda S, Cavalcante F, Axelband F, et al. Involvement of the Gi/o/cGMP/PKG pathway in the AT2-mediated inhibition of outer cortex proximal tubule Na+-ATPase by Ang-(1–7). *Biochem J* 2006;395: 183–190.

[64] Albiston AL, McDowall SG, Matsacos D, et al. Evidence that the angiotensin IV (AT(4)) receptor is the enzyme insulin-regulated aminopeptidase. *J Biol Chem* 2001;276:48623–48626.

[65] Weber KT, Brilla CG. Pathological hypertrophy and cardiac interstitium. Fibrosis and renin–angiotensin–aldosterone system. *Circulation* 1991;83:1849–1865.

[66] Steckelings UM, Kaschina E, Unger T. The AT2 receptor-A matter of love and hate. *Peptides* 2005;26:1401–1409.

[67] Funke-Kaiser H, Reinemund J, Steckelings UM, et al. Adapter proteins and promoter regulation of the angiotensin II type 2 receptor—implications for cardiac pathophysiology. *J Renin Angiotensin Aldosterone Syst* 2010;11:7–17.

[68] Seyedi N, Xu X, Nasjletti A, et al. Coronary kinin generation mediates nitric oxide release after angiotensin receptor stimulation. *Hypertension* 1995; 26:164–170.

[69] Nouet S, Nahmias C. Signal transduction from the angiotensin II AT2 receptor. *Trends Endocrinol Metab* 2006;11:1–6.

[70] Kaschina E, Grzesiak A, Li J, Foryst-Ludwig A, et al. Angiotensin II type 2 receptor stimulation: a novel option of therapeutic interference with the renin-angiotensin system in myocardial infarction? *Circulation* 2008;118:2523–2532.

[71] Rompe F, Artuc M, Hallberg A, et al. Direct angiotensin II type 2 receptor stimulation acts anti-inflammatory through epoxyeicosatrienoic acid and inhibition of nuclear factor {kappa}B. *Hypertension* 2010;55:924–931.

[72] Dias-Peixoto MF, Santos RA, Gomes ER, et al. Molecular mechanisms involved in the angiotensin-(1–7)/Mas signaling pathway in cardiomyocytes. *Hypertension* 2008;52:542–548.

[73] Fraga-Silva RA, Pinheiro SV, Gonc¸alves AC, et al. The antithrombotic effect of angiotensin-(1–7) involves mas-mediated NO release from platelets. *Mol Med* 2008;14:28–35.

[74] da Silveira KD, Coelho FM, Vieira AT, et al. Anti-inflammatory effects of the activation of the angiotensin-(1–7) receptor, MAS, in experimental models of arthritis. *J Immunol* 2010;185:5569–5576.

[75] Savergnini SQ, Beiman M, Lautner RQ, et al. Vascular relaxation, antihypertensive effect, and cardioprotection of a novel peptide agonist of the MAS receptor. *Hypertension* 2010;56:112–120.

[76] Cozzari C, Angeletti PU, Lazar J, et al. Separation of isorenin activity from nerve growth factor (NGF) activity in mouse submaxillary gland extracts. *Biochem Pharmacol* 1973; 22: 1321–1327.
[77] Hirose S, Ohsawa T, Inagami T, et al. Brain renin from bovine anterior pituitary. Isolation and properties. *J Biol Chem* 1982; 257: 6316–6321.
[78] Tada M, Fukamizu A, Seo MS, et al. Renin expression in the kidney and brain is reciprocally controlled by captopril. *Biochem Biophys Res Commun* 1989; 159: 1065–1071.
[79] Mann JF, Rascher W, Scho¨mig A, et al. Contribution of the sympathetic nervous system to the centrally-induced pressor action of angiotensin II in rats. *Clin Exp Pharmacol Physiol* 1982; 9: 193–201.
[80] Sumners C, Phillips MI. Central injection of angiotensin II alters catecholamine activity in rat brain. *Am J Physiol* 1983; 244: R257–R263.
[81] Sasaki S, Takeda K, Okajima H, et al. Pressor responses to intracisternal injection of hypertonic NaCl in rats. *J Cardiovasc Pharmacol* 1984; 6: 349–354.
[82] Bun˜ ag RD, Miyajima E. Sympathetic hyperactivity elevates blood pressure during acute cerebroventricular infusions of hypertonic salt in rats. *J Cardiovasc Pharmacol* 1984; 6: 844–851.
[83] Sakamoto M, Nishimura M, Takahashi H. Brain atrial natriuretic peptide family abolishes cardiovascular haemodynamic alterations caused by hypertonic saline in rats. *Clin Exp Pharmacol Physiol* 1999; 26: 684–690.
[84] Cai H, Harrison DG. Endothelial dysfunction in cardiovascular diseases: the role of oxidant stress. *Circ Res*. 2000; 87:840–844.
[85] Laursen JB, Somers M, Kurz S, et al. Endothelial regulation of vasomotion in apoE-deficient mice : Implications for interactions between peroxynitrite and tetrahydrobiopterin. *Circulation*. 2001; 103:1282–1288.
[86] Munzel T, Daiber A, Ullrich V, et al. Vascular consequences of endothelial nitric oxide synthase uncoupling for the activity and expression of the soluble guanylyl cyclase and the cGMPdependent protein kinase. *Arterioscler Thromb Vasc Biol*. 2005; 25:1551–1557.
[87] Thomas SR, Chen K, Keaney JF Jr. Hydrogen peroxide activates endothelial nitric-oxide synthase through coordinated phosphorylation and dephosphorylation via a phosphoinositide 3-kinasedependent signaling pathway. *J Biol Chem*. 2002; 277:6017–6024.
[88] Drummond GR, Cai H, Davis ME, et al.Transcriptional and posttranscriptional regulation of endothelial nitric oxide synthase expression by hydrogen peroxide. *Circ Res*. 2000; 86:347–354.
[89] Stocker R, Keaney JF Jr. The role of oxidative modifications in atherosclerosis. Physiol Rev. 2004; 84:1381–1478.
[90] Chen K, Thomas SR, Keaney JF Jr. Beyond LDL oxidation: ROS in vascular signal transduction. *Free Radic Biol Med*. 2003; 35:117–132.
[91] Harrison DG, Gongora MC. Oxidative stress and hypertension. *Med Clin North Am*. 2009;93:621–635.
[92] Hoch NE, Guzik TJ, Chen W, et al. Regulation of T-cell function by endogenously produced angiotensin II. *Am J Physiol Regul Integr Comp Physiol*. 2009; 296:R208–R216.

[93] Miyagawa K, Ohashi M, Yamashita S, et al. Increased oxidative stress impairs endothelial modulation of contractions in arteries from spontaneously hypertensive rats. *J Hypertens*. 2007; 25:415–421.

[94] Friedman J, Peleg E, Kagan T, et al. Oxidative stress in hypertensive,diabetic, and diabetic hypertensive rats. *Am J Hypertens.* 2003; 16:1049–1052.

[95] Trolliet MR, Rudd MA, Loscalzo J. Oxidative stress and renal dysfunction in salt-sensitive hypertension. Kidney Blood Press Res. 2001; 24:116–123.

[96] Koga Y, Hirooka Y, Araki S, et al. High salt intake enhances blood pressure increase during development of hypertension via oxidative stress in rostral ventrolateral medulla of spontaneously hypertensive rats. *Hypertens Res*. 2008; 31:2075–2083.

[97] Lerman LO, Nath KA, Rodriguez-Porcel M, et al. Increased oxidative stress in experimental renovascular hypertension. *Hypertension*. 2001; 37:541–546.

[98] Oliveira-Sales EB, Nishi EE, Carillo BA, et al. Oxidative stress in the sympathetic premotor neurons contributes to sympathetic activation in renovascular hypertension. *Am J Hypertens*. 2009; 22:484–492.

[99] Dobrian AD, Davies MJ, Schriver SD, et al. Oxidative stress in a rat model of obesity-induced hypertension. *Hypertension*. 2001; 37:554–560.

[100] Lopez-Campistrous A, Hao L, Xiang W, et al. Mitochondrial dysfunction in the hypertensive rat brain: respiratory complexes exhibit assembly defects in hypertension. *Hypertension*. 2008; 51:412–419.

[101] Callera GE, Tostes RC, Yogi A, et al. Endothelin-1-induced oxidative stress in DOCA-salt hypertension involves NADPH-oxidase-independent mechanisms. *Clin Sci* (Lond).2006; 110:243–253.

[102] Tinoy JK, Michael EW. Natural Antioxidants and Hypertension: Promise and Challenges. *Cardiovasc Ther*. 2010 ; 28: e20–e32.

[103] London G, Marchais S, Guerin A. Arterial stiffness and function in end-stage renal disease. *Adv Chron Kidney Dis*. 2004; 11:202–209.

[104] World Health Organization–International Society of Hypertension guidelines for the management of hypertension. Guidelines Subcommittee. *J Hypertens*. 1999;17:151–183.

[105] Oparil S. High blood pressure. In: Goldman L, Bennett JC, eds. Cecil Textbook of Medicine: 21st Century Edition. Philadelphia, Pa: WB Saunders; 1999.

[106] Puddey IB, Cox K. Exercise lowers blood pressure2sometimes? Or did Pheidippides have hypertension? J Hypertens. 1995;13:1229 –1233. Editorial.

[107] Arkwright PD, Beilin LJ, Rouse I, Armstrong BK, Vandongen R. Effects of alcohol use and other aspects of lifestyle on blood pressure levels and prevalence of hypertension in a working population. *Circulation*. 1982; 66:60–66.

[108] Beilin LJ, Puddey IB, Burke V. Alcohol and hypertension: kill or cure? *J Hum Hypertens*. 1996;10(suppl 2):S1–S5.

[109] Puddey IB, Beilin LJ, Rakic V. Alcohol, hypertension and the cardiovascular system: a critical appraisal. *Addict Biol*. 1997;2:159 –170.

[110] MacMahon S. Alcohol consumption and hypertension. *Hypertension*. 1987;9:111–121.

[111] McCarron DA, Oparil S, Chait A, Haynes RB, Kris-Etherton P, Stern JS, Resnick LM, Clark S, Morris CD, Hatton DC, Metz JA, McMahon M, Holcomb S, Snyder GW, Pi-Sunyer FX. Nutritional management of cardiovascular risk factors: a randomized clinical trial. *Arch Intern Med*. 1997;157:169 –177.

[112] Svetkey LP, Simons-Morton D, Vollmer WM, Appel LJ, Conlin PR, Ryan DH, Ard J, Kennedy BM, for the DASH Research Group. Effects of dietary patterns on blood pressure: subgroup analysis of the Dietary Approaches to Stop Hypertension (DASH) randomized clinical trial. *Arch Intern Med.* 1999;159:285–293.
[113] Moore TJ, Appel LJ, Bray GA, Svetkey LP, Vollmer WM. More salt, please: the DASH Steering Committee. Science. 1998;282:1049 –1051. Letter.
[114] Oparil S, Calhoun DA. High blood pressure. *Sci Am Med.* 1997;1:1–14.
[115] Kotchen TA, McCarron DA, for the Nutrition Group. Dietary electrolytes and blood pressure. *Circulation.* 1998;98:613– 617.
[116] Kassirer JP, Harrington JT. Fending off the potassium pushers. *N Engl J Med.* 1985;312:785–787. Editorial.
[117] Burt VL, Whelton P, Roccella EJ, Brown C, Cutler JA, Higgins M, Horan MJ, Labarthe D. Prevalence of hypertension in the US adult population: results from the Third National Health and Nutrition Examination Survey, 1988–1991. *Hypertension.* 1995;25:305–313.
[118] Oscar AC, Suzanne O. Essential Hypertension : Part II: Treatment. *Circulation.* 2000;101:446-453
[199] Paulis L, Unger T. Novel therapeutic targets for hypertension. *Nat Rev Cardiol* 2010;7:431–441.
[200] Krum H, Schlaich M, Sobotka P, et al. Novel procedure- and device-based strategies in the management of systemic hypertension. *Eur Heart J* 2011;32:537–544.
[201] Kurtz TW. Beyond the classic angiotensin-receptor-blocker profile. *Nat Clin Pract Cardiovasc Med* 2008;5:S19–S26.
[202] Kappert K, Tsuprykov O, Kaufmann J, et al. Chronic treatment with losartan results in sufficient serum levels of the metabolite EXP3179 for PPARgamma activation. *Hypertension* 2009;54:738–743.
[203] Gradman AH, Vivas Y. New drugs for hypertension: what do they offer? *Curr Hypertens Rep* 2006;8:425–432.
[204. Dietz R, Dechend R, Yu CM, et al. Effects of the direct renin inhibitor aliskiren and atenolol alone or in combination in patients with hypertension. *J Renin Angiotensin Aldosterone Syst* 2008;9:163–175.
[205] Schmieder RE, Philipp T, Guerediaga J, et al. Long-term antihypertensive efficacy and safety of the oral direct renin inhibitor aliskiren: a 12-month randomized, double-blind comparator trial with hydrochlorothiazide. *Circulation* 2009;119: 417–425.
[206] Andersen K, Weinberger MH, Egan B, et al. Comparative efficacy and safety of aliskiren, an oral direct renin inhibitor, and ramipril in hypertension: a 6-month, randomized, double-blind trial. *J Hypertens* 2008;26:589–599.
[207] Stanton A, Jensen C, Nussberger J, et al. Blood pressure lowering in essential hypertension with an oral renin inhibitor, aliskiren. *Hypertension* 2003;42: 1137–1143.
[208] Schefe JH, Neumann C, Goebel M, et al. Prorenin engages the (pro)renin receptor like rennin and both ligand activities are unopposed by aliskiren. *J Hypertens* 2008;26: 1787–1794.
[209] Huang Y, Wongamorntham S, Kasting J, et al. Renin increases mesangial cell transforming growth factor-beta1 and matrix proteins through receptor-mediated, angiotensin II-independent mechanisms. *Kidney Int* 2006;69:105–113.

[210] Feldt S, Maschke U, Dechend R, et al. The putative (pro)rennin receptor blocker HRP fails to prevent (pro)renin signaling. *J Am Soc Nephrol* 2008;19:743–748.

[211] Susic D, Zhou X, Frohlich ED, et al. Cardiovascular effects of prorenin blockade in genetically spontaneously hypertensive rats on normal and high-salt diet. *Am J Physiol Heart Circ Physiol* 2008;295:H1117–H1121.

[212] Dive V, Chang CF, Yiotakis A, et al. Inhibition of zinc metallopeptidases in cardiovascular disease—from unity to trinity, or duality? *Curr Pharm Des* 2009; 15:3606–3621.

[213] Campbell DJ. Vasopeptidase inhibition: a double-edged sword? *Hypertension* 2003;41:383–389.

[214] d'Uscio LV, Quaschning T, Burnett JC Jr, et al. Vasopeptidase inhibition prevents endothelial dysfunction of resistance arteries in salt-sensitive hypertension in comparison with single ACE inhibition. *Hypertension* 2001;37:28–33.

[215] Kostis JB, Packer M, Black HR, et al. Omapatrilat and enalapril in patients with hypertension: the Omapatrilat Cardiovascular Treatment vs. Enalapril (OCTAVE) trial. *Am J Hypertens* 2004;17:103–111.

[216] Nishizaka MK, Zaman MA, Calhoun DA. Efficacy of low-dose spironolactone in subjects with resistant hypertension. *Am J Hypertens* 2003;16:925–930.

[217] Mehdi UF, Adams-Huet B, Raskin P, et al. Addition of angiotensin receptor blockade or mineralocorticoid antagonism to maximal angiotensinconverting enzyme inhibition in diabetic nephropathy. *J Am Soc Nephrol* 2009; 20:2641–2650.

[218] Pitt B, Remme W, Zannad F, et al. Eplerenone Post-Acute Myocardial Infarction Heart Failure Efficacy and Survival Study Investigators. Eplerenone, a selective aldosterone blocker, in patients with left ventricular dysfunction after myocardial infarction. *N Engl J Med* 2003;348:1309–1321.

[219] Schmidt BM, Schmieder RE. Aldosterone-induced cardiac damage: focus on blood pressure independent effects. *Am J Hypertens* 2003;16:80–86.

[220] Gaddam K, Pimenta E, Thomas SJ, et al. Spironolactone reduces severity of obstructive sleep apnoea in patients with resistant hypertension: a preliminary report. *J Hum Hypertens* 2010;24:532–537.

[221] Fiebeler A, Nussberger J, Shagdarsuren E, et al. Aldosterone synthase inhibitor ameliorates angiotensin II-induced organ damage. *Circulation* 2005;111:3087–3094.

[222] Huang BS, White RA, Jeng AY, et al. Role of central nervous system aldosterone synthase and mineralocorticoid receptors in salt-induced hypertension in Dahl salt-sensitive rats. *Am J Physiol Regul Integr Comp Physiol* 2009;296: [R994–R1000.

[223] Lea WB, Kwak ES, Luther JM, et al. Aldosterone antagonism or synthase inhibition reduces end-organ damage induced by treatment with angiotensin and high salt. *Kidney Int* 2009;75: 936–944.

[224] Feldstein C, Romero C. Role of endothelins in hypertension. *Am J Ther* 2007;14: 147–153.

[225] Bakris GL, Lindholm LH, Black HR, et al. Divergent results using clinic and ambulatory blood pressures: report of a darusentan-resistant hypertension trial. *Hypertension* 2010;56: 824–830.

[226] Sica DA. Endothelin receptor antagonism: what does the future hold? *Hypertension* 2008;52:460–461.

[227] Xu J, Li G, Wang P, et al. Renalase is a novel, soluble monoamine oxidase that regulates cardiac function and blood pressure. *J Clin Invest* 2005;115:1275–1280.
[228] Li G, Xu J,Wang P, et al. Catecholamines regulate the activity, secretion, and synthesis of renalase. *Circulation* 2008;117: 1277–1282.
[229] Desir GV. Role of renalase in the regulation of blood pressure and the renal dopamine system. *Opin Nephrol Hypertens* 2011;20:31–36.
[230] Zhao Q, Fan Z, He J, et al. Renalase gene is a novel susceptibility gene for essential hypertension: a two-stage association study in northern Han Chinese population. *J Mol Med* 2007;85:877–885.
[237] Huentelman MJ, Grobe JL, Vazquez J, et al. Protection from angiotensin II-induced cardiac hypertrophy and fibrosis by systemic lentiviral delivery of ACE2 in rats. *Exp Physiol* 2005;90:783–790.
[238] Li H, Gao Y, Grobe JL, Raizada MK, et al. Potentiation of the antihypertensive action of losartan by peripheral overexpression of the ANG II type 2 receptor. *Am J Physiol Heart Circ Physiol* 2007;292:H727–H735.
[239] Sun H, Zhang L, Wang A, et al. Prolonged hypotensive effect of human tissue kallikrein gene delivery and recombinant enzyme administration in spontaneous hypertension rats. *Exp Mol Med* 2004;36:23–27.
[240] Vaneckova´ I, Kopkan L, Huskova´ Z, et al. AT1 receptor antisense therapy transiently lowers blood pressure in Ren-2 transgenic rats. *Vascul Pharmacol* 2007;47:63–67.
[241] Landa MS, Garcı´a SI, Schuman ML, et al. Knocking down the diencephalic thyrotropin-releasing hormone precursor gene normalizes obesity-induced hypertension in the rat. *Am J Physiol Endocrinol Metab* 2007;292:E1388–E1394.
[242] Ambu¨hl PM, Tissot AC, Fulurija A, et al. A vaccine for hypertension based on virus-like particles: preclinical efficacy and phase I safety and immunogenicity. *J Hypertens* 2007;25:63–72.
[243] Tissot AC, Maurer P, Nussberger J, et al. Effect of immunization against angiotensin II with CYT006-AngQb on ambulatory blood pressure: a double-blind, randomised, placebo-controlled phase IIa study. *Lancet* 2008;371: 821–827.
[244] Oneda B, Ortega KC, Gusma˜o JL, et al. Sympathetic nerve activity is decreased during device-guided slow breathing. *Hypertens Res* 2010; 33:708–712.
[245] Parati G, Carretta R. Device-guided slow breathing as a non-pharmacological approach to antihypertensive treatment: efficacy, problems and perspectives. *J Hypertens* 2007;25:57–61.
[246] Schlaich MP, Sobotka PA, Krum H, et al. Renal denervation as a therapeutic approach for hypertension: novel implications for an old concept. *Hypertension* 2009;54:1195–1201.
[247] Symplicity HTN-2 Investigators, Esler MD, Krum H, et al. Renal sympathetic denervation in patients with treatment-resistant hypertension (The Symplicity HTN-2 Trial): a randomized controlled trial. *Lancet* 2010;376:1903–1909.
[248] Doumas M, Douma S. Renal denervation: the jury is still out. Lancet 2010;376: 1878–1880.
[249] Sica DA, Lohmeier TE. Baroreflex activation for the treatment of hypertension: principles and practice. *Expert Rev Med Devices* 2006;3:595–601.
[250] Scheffers IJ, Kroon AA, Tordoir JH, et al. Rheos baroreflex hypertension therapy system to treat resistant hypertension. *Expert Rev Med Devices* 2008; 5:33–39.

[251] Sica DA. Rationale for fixed-dose combinations in the treatment of hypertension: the cycle repeats. *Drugs* 2002;62:443–462.

[252] Thomas U, Ludovit P, Domenic AS. Therapeutic perspectives in hypertension: novel means for renin–angiotensin–aldosterone system modulation and emerging device-based approaches. *European Heart Journal* 2011; 32:2739–2747.

In: Arterial Hypertension
Editors: Marten Vosler and Siemen Weber

ISBN: 978-1-62417-852-8
© 2013 Nova Science Publishers, Inc.

Chapter 4

Arterial Hypertension: Influence of Sex Hormones

Roger Lyrio dos Santos,[1] Wender do Nascimento Rouver,[2] IzabelaFacco Caliman,[2] Aline Zandonadi Lamas,[2] Fabrício Bragança da Silva[2] and Sônia Alves Gouvea[1]

[1]Department of Physiological Sciences
[2]Postgraduate Program in Physiological Sciences,
Federal University of Espírito Santo, Vitória, Brazil

Abstract

Sex hormones are steroids derived from cholesterol, which have numerous biological functions on reproductive organs, glands from these organs and on important systems of our organism controlling or modulating various functions such as reproduction, growth and metabolism. Moreover, the sex hormones are able to modulate blood pressure by acting on important systems as cardiovascular, renal and neural. These hormones can have either complementary or antagonistic actions. Indeed, it has been described in the technical literature that the actions of testosterone are contrary to the estrogen in the regulation of blood pressure. Estrogen alone or combined with progesterone has been associated with decreased blood pressure, whereas testosterone can raise blood pressure by stimulating the renin-angiotensin-aldosterone system. The effects of testosterone in the development of cardiovascular disease (CVD) are contradictory. While some researchers suggest positive effect, others indicate negative actions of testosterone. It has been reported that androgen deprivation in adult men impaired endothelium-dependent relaxation and promoted the progression of atherosclerosis. Nevertheless, many other clinical and epidemiological studies have also reported that testosterone inhibits CVD development. Another evidence about the benefits of the male sex hormone is laid down when we assess the effects of induced hypogonadism on hypertension by analyzing large artery stiffening in men. Studies have shown that after three months of induced hypogonadism diastolic pressure is elevated, along with mean pulse pressure. Similarly, estrogen showed protective effects on vascular function and heart failure, which are related to the prevention of arterial hypertension. Estrogens can promote vasodilation and lower BP by different mechanisms as their direct actions on blood vessels, which physiologically stimulate the release of endothelium-derived vasodilator factors as well as modification of vasoconstrictor factors and inhibition of the renin-angiotensin system. Although the cardioprotective effects of estrogen are widely appreciated, little is known about the effects of progesterone, which is commonly used in hormone replacement therapy (HRT). Progesterone has both vasodilatory and vasoconstrictive effects in the vasculature depending on location of the vessel and level of exposure. Indeed, progesterone at physiological levels can inhibit the production of endothelin-1, but at supraphysiological levels, it inhibits endothelium-independent relaxation. Despite the alleged benefits of estrogen and progesterone on cardiovascular disease, the use of these hormones to postmenopausal women for HRT are still controversial. In addition, the negative findings of Heart and Estrogen/progestin Replacement Study (HERS) I and II and Women's Health Initiative (WHI) studies on HRT in postmenopausal women, such as stroke, venous thromboembolic disease and deep vein thrombosis have shaken our previous ideas that HRT was protective. Thus, other therapies being tested in hormone replacement as the selective estrogen receptor modulator (SERMs) that, like estrogen, may induce endothelium-dependent acute vasodilation resulting in lowering of blood pressure. However, the mechanisms through which sex hormones modulate the blood pressure have not been fully elucidated. Therefore, the characterization of those could lead to a better understanding of hypertension in women and men, and perhaps to improved forms of therapy. In this chapter we will be a discussing the potential mechanisms through which male and female sex hormones may regulate the blood pressure as well as the cellular, biochemical and molecular pathways by which sex hormones may modify the effects of hypertension on the cardiovascular system.

1. Introduction

Numerous studies have shown that female human beings exhibit lower blood pressure levels over much of their life span compared with their age-matched counterparts. Steroid hormones regulate a wide variety of events in the human bod, as blood pressure levels (BP), an important factor in the development of hypertension and coronary artery disease, some of the most common cardiovascular diseases in the industrialized world (Qiao et al., 2008; Wang et al., 2012). This sexual dimorphism is apparent in human beings as well as most, if not all, mammals. However, after the onset of menopause blood pressure levels in women increase and become similar to those in men, suggesting an important role of sex hormones in the regulation of blood pressure (Miller, 2010; Maric-Bilkan and Manigrasso., 2012). In fact, both estrogens and androgens have been implicated in the development of cardiovascular disease and hypertension, with estrogens, in general, being protective and androgens being bidirectional.

Although some studies suggest that testosterone may exert deleterious effects on the vascular wall by enhancing vascular tone through acute or chronic mechanisms (McCredie el al., 1998), considerable evidence now suggests that testosterone and other androgens have protective effects on cardiovascular and may play important roles in the acute regulation of vascular function (Nettleship et al.,2009).

Indeed, studies have demonstrated that testosterone exerts beneficial effects on cardiovascular function by inducing rapid vasorelaxation of vascular smooth muscle (Traish et al., 2009).

Although the exact mechanisms by which sex hormones contribute to the regulation of cardiovascular function and blood pressure are still being investigated, there is increasing evidence that modulating the activity of locally active hormone systems is one of the major mechanisms of sex hormone actions in target organs, including the vasculature and kidneys (Orshal and Khalil., 2004; Maric-Bilkan and Manigrasso., 2012). Estrogen, progesterone, and testosterone receptors have been identified in blood vessels and may induced stimulation of the endothelium-dependent mechanisms of vascular relaxation and inhibition of the mechanisms of vascular smooth muscle contraction, which contribute to the gender differences in vascular tone and may represent potential beneficial vascular effects of hormone replacement therapy during natural and surgically induced deficiencies of gonadal hormones (Orshal and Khalil., 2004; Qiao et al., 2008; Cutini et al., 2012).

2. Biosynthesis and Secretion of Sex Hormones

The biosynthetic pathways in all endocrine organs that form steroid hormones are similar, however the organs differing only in the enzyme systems they contain (figure 2). Estrogen is the main female sex hormone in both humans and animal models. It is produced in the granulosa cells of the ovarian cortex through the conversion of androgen precursors by the aromatase enzyme, which in turn is modulated by the hormonal hypothalamic-pituitary axis. Soon, testosterone is a key intermediate in both women and men, being converted to estrogen by the action of aromatase and to the more potent androgen, dihydrotestosterone, by 5- α reductase. In women estradiol is the main form of circulating estrogen, and circulating levels of testosterone are relatively low.

A key point, though, is that circulating levels of hormones may not reflect those at the tissue level, as both aromatase and 5-α reductase can be found in a number of tissues, including blood vessels. For example, in bone, testosterone is converted to 17β- estradiol by aromatase; estradiol then acts locally to promote mineralization and prevent osteoporosis (Virginia et al 2008).

The biosynthesis of ovarian aromatases and hence estrogen production are under the control of the gonadotropins, FSH and LH (figure 1). These processes are controlled by the size and frequency of GnRH pulses, as well as by feedback from estrogens.

In females the frequency of the pulses varies during the menstrual cycle, and there is a large surge of GnRH just before ovulation.

Moreover, estrogens may exert autoregulatory effects on their own production via positive feedback mechanisms (Zhuang et al., 1982). Estrogen has a bimodal effect on the hypothalamus with both an inhibitory and stimulatory influence on GnRH secretion. The stimulatory effect of estrogen is seen at the end of the follicular phase where estrogen triggers the preovulatory GnRH surge (Sarkar et al., 1976).

The ability of estrogen to induce a surge declines with age in female rodents and women (Wise, 1982; Shaw et al., 2011) This appears to be due in large part to a decrease in estrogen induction of GnRH neurons, particularly in rodents (Downs and Wise, 2009), although a decline in pituitary responsiveness to GnRH contributing to attenuated luteinizing hormone (LH) surges has also been proposed (Shaw et al., 2009).

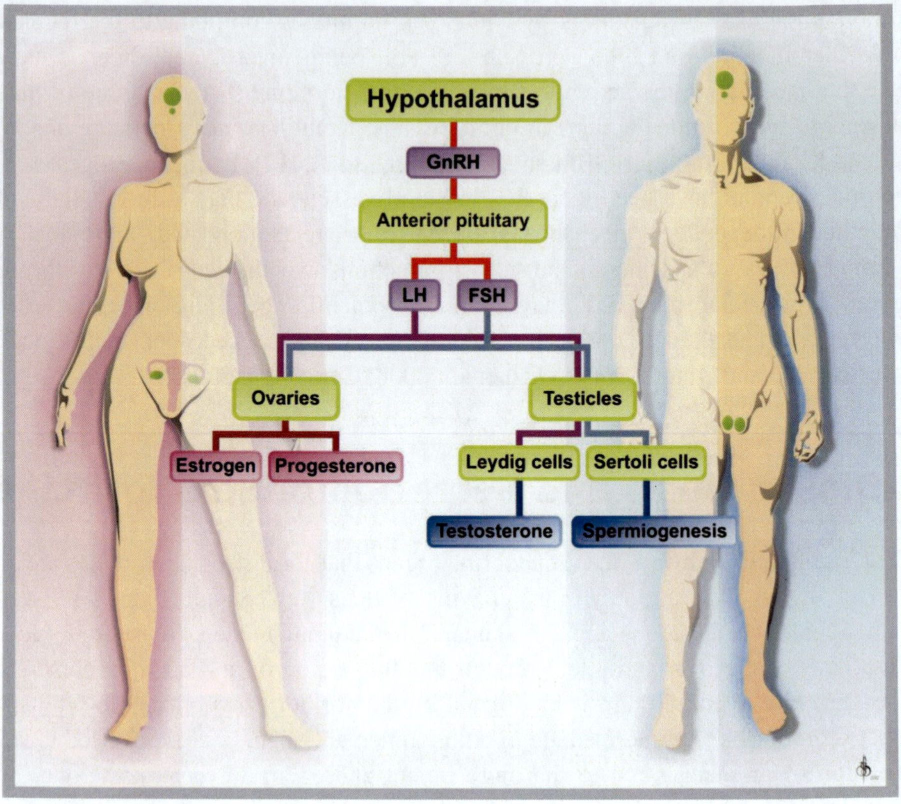

Figure 1. Overview of the action of gonadotropins in men and women.

As estrogen, most of the synthesis of progesterone also occurs in the ovary. After follicle rupture and release of the ovum, these granulosa cells mature to form the corpus luteum, which is responsible for secretion of progesterone and estrogen in the latter part of the cycle.

In the human, if fertilization does not occur within 1 to 2 days, the corpus luteum will continue to enlarge for 10 –12 days followed by regression of the gland and concomitant cessation of estrogen and progesterone release. If fertilization occurs, the corpus luteum will continue to grow and function for the first 2 to 3 months of pregnancy. After this time it will slowly regress as the placenta assumes the role of hormonal biosynthesis for the maintenance of pregnancy.

The principal hormone of the testes is testosterone, it is a C_{19} steroid with an -OH group in the 17 position, synthesized from cholesterol in the Leydig cells and is also formed from androstenedione secreted by the adrenal cortex. In the Leydig cells, the 11- and 21-hydroxylases found in the adrenal cortex are absent, but 17α-hydroxylase is present. The first step to biosynthesis of testosterone, as well as to the other steroids, is the conversion of cholesterol to pregnenolone by cholesterol desmolase (figure 2). Then pregnenolone is hydroxylated in the 17 position and subjected to side chain cleavage to form dehydroepiandrosterone, that is converted into androstenedione.

In addition, pregnenolone can be converted in progesterone that will form androstenedione, but this pathway is less prominent in humans. Finally, androstenedione is converted to testosterone (Weiss et al., 2008).

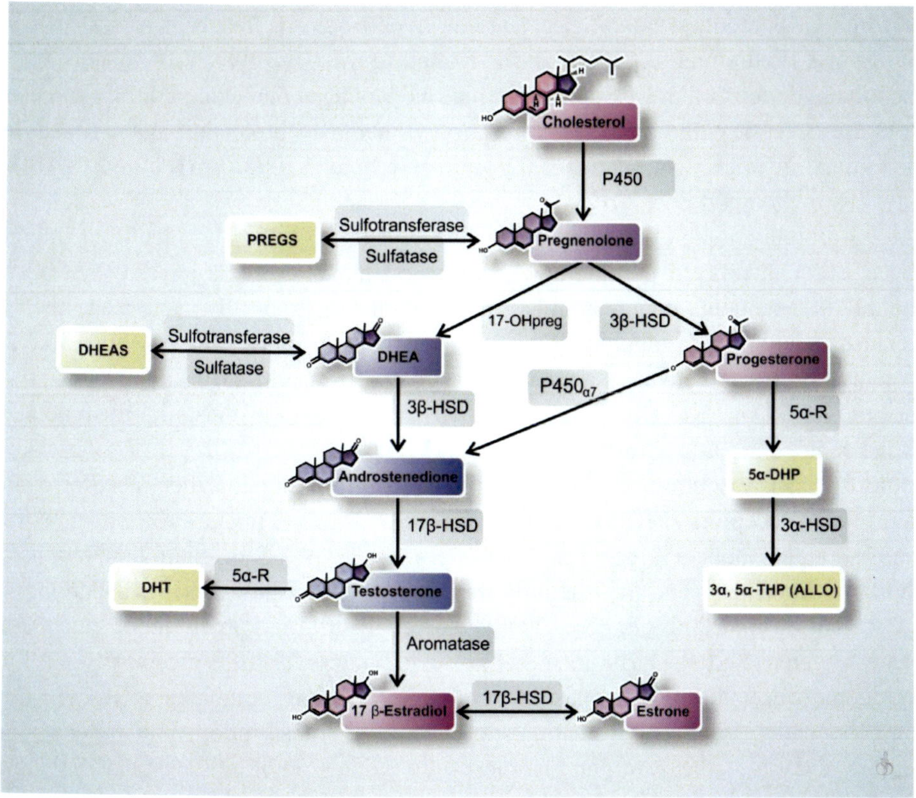

Figure 2. Biosynthesis of steroid hormones.

The secretion of testosterone is under the control of LH, and the mechanism by which LH stimulates the Leydig cells involves increased formation of cAMP via the G protein-coupled LH receptor and Gs. Cyclic AMP increases the formation of cholesterol from cholesterol esters and the conversion of cholesterol to pregnenolone via the activation of protein kinase A. Nevertheless, the testosterone secretion rate is 4-9 mg/d (13.9-31.33 µmol/d) in normal adult males. Small amounts of testosterone are also secreted in females, probably from the ovary but possibly from the adrenal as well (Pathirana et al., 2012).

3. Mechanism of Action of Sex Hormones

The estrogen's effects in target tissues occur mainly by activating one or all three estrogen receptors, estrogen receptor (ER) α, ERβ and G protein–coupled ER (GPER), the latter being also known as G-protein coupled receptor 30 (GPR30) and as the membrane estrogen receptor (mER) (Zhu et al 2002; Barton et al 2011). These receptors are largest distribute in tissues of both sexes, including cardiovascular and reproductive systems, liver, brain and bone.

ERα and β are found both in associations with the plasma membrane, in the cytoplasm and in the nucleus (Knowlton and Lee, 2012). Some of the known functions of ERα are related to activation of eNOS (Dessy et al., 2010; Fleming, 2010), prevention of VSMC proliferation (Takahashi et al., 2003) and to inhibit increase in medial thickness (Pare et al.,

2002), while ERβ reduces pathological cardiac hypertrophy (Fliegner et al., 2010), inhibit cardiac fibrosis (Pedram et al., 2010) and is related to the development of sustained systolic and diastolic hypertension in ERβ-deficient mice as they age (Zhu et al., 2002). Both estrogen receptors are necessary and sufficient for estrogen-mediated protection against measures of vascular injury in mice (Zhu et al., 2002) and may activate PI3K, AKT and MAP kinase pathways (Knowlton and Lee, 2012).

The G-protein-coupled estrogen receptor (GPER), a recently identified membrane associated ER, can relaxed porcine aortic rings and human coronary artery VSMCs in an endothelial independent manner and your activation especially activated the large-conductance calcium and voltage activated potassium channels (BK_{Ca}) (Yu et al., 2011). Additionally GPER can activate the nonnuclear protective response (PI3-kinase, Akt, etc.) via a truncated 36 kDa ERα (Kang et al., 2010) and attenuate diastolic dysfunction and ventricular remodeling after ovariectomized rats (Wang et al., 2012).

Some estrogen's actions have been evoked by its binding to other receptors, such as estrogen related receptors (ERRs). These receptors are orphan nuclear receptors, with three isoforms — alpha, beta and gamma. The ERRs are involved in energy metabolism and mitochondrial biogenesis and their activity depends on coactivator proteins (Schreiber et al., 2003; Bookout et al., 2006; Giguère, 2008). However, little is known about the interaction between estrogen and ERRs and some other possible binders for these receptors.

Estrogen diffuses through the plasma membrane and forms complexes with cytosolic and nuclear ERs, which bind to chromatin, stimulate gene transcription, and induce genomic effects. For example, the estrogen deficiency in young adult rats resulted in increased expression of a number of pro-inflammatory genes in the heart including L-selectin, calpain, TNF, iNOS and fibronectin (Hamilton et al., 2007). Furthermore, estrogen also binds to signal-generating ERs on the plasma membrane of vascular cells and induces rapid nongenomic endothelium-dependent and -independent signaling cascades (PI3K and Akt, as well as ERK 1/2, JNK and p38) (Wu et al., 2011) and vascular effects (Qiao et al, 2008).

Progesterone (P4) effects, in turn, are mediated by binding to the nuclear progesterone receptor (PR) (Scarpin et al., 2009). Receptors for progesterone are expressed as two distinct isoforms, PR-A and PR-B, which arise from a single gene (Conneely et al., 2002) (7), and are present in various human tissues including the uterus, mammary gland, brain, pancreas, bone, ovary, testes, and tissues of the lower urinary tract. The ubiquitous expression of PR highlights the widespread physiological effects that progesterone can exert in a variety of organs throughout the body (Scarpin et al., 2009).

The general pathway of P4 inducible PR-mediated gene transcription has been well characterized. P4 binding induces a conformational change(s) in PR that promote dissociation from a multi-protein chaperone complex, homodimerization and binding to specific progesterone response elements (PREs) within the promoter of target genes. DNA bound receptors increase or decrease rates of gene transcription by influencing recruitment of RNA polymerase II to the initiation site. Through protein–protein interaction, hormone activated PR recruits coactivators that serve as essential intermediates for transmitting signals from the receptor to the transcription initiation complex. Coactivators facilitate transcription initiation through protein interactions with components of the general transcription machinery and by promoting local remodeling of chromatin at specific promoters (Leonhardt et al., 2003).

A new class of progesterone receptors located at the plasma membrane was found primarily in spotted sea trout ovaries (Zhu et al., 2003) and subsequently detected in human tissues (Karteris et al., 2006). Membrane receptors for progesterone (mPR) has three isoforms (mPRα, mPRβ, and mPRγ) that are structurally unrelated to nuclear steroid receptors, but instead has features typical of G protein-coupled receptors. The non-genomic mechanisms of action of the mPRs are typically coupled to the inhibitory G-protein Gα_i, whereby progesterone stimulation decreases cAMP synthesis that is sensitive to pertussis toxin inhibition (Zhu et al., 2003). mPR stimulation also causes activating phosphorylations of the mitogen activated protein kinases ERK1/2 and JNK1/2 (Karteris et al., 2006).

All three isoforms of mPRs shown to bind progesterone with high affinity, while not interacting with either synthetic progestins or anti-progestins (Thomas et al., 2007).

The androgen receptor (AR) exists in two forms, ARα and ARβ, which have distinct tissue expression patterns (Wilson and McPhaul, 1996). Sex differences in the distribution and abundance of AR have been demonstrated in a variety of tissues including vascular smooth muscle cells and endothelial cells (Negro-Vilar, 1999). Like other steroids, testosterone binds to an intracellular receptor, and the receptor-steroid complex then binds to DNA in the nucleus, facilitating transcription of various genes. In some target cells, testosterone is converted to dihydrotestosterone (DHT) by 5α- reductase and DHT binds to the same intracellular receptor as testosterone. Testosterone-receptor complexes are less stable than DHT-receptor complexes in target cells, and they conform less well to the DNA-binding state. Thus, DHT formation is a way of amplifying the action of testosterone in target tissues. In addition to genomic effect, testosterone can induce non-genomic effect by membrane receptors. The non-genomic effects are rapidly produced, do not require the association of androgen receptors to DNA. These effects involve the activation of various signaling pathways, including calcium, protein kinase A, protein kinase C, and mitogen-activated protein kinase (MAPK)(Bhasin and Jasuja, 2009).

Thus, both the male sex hormones as the female are able to act through genomic and no-genomic mechanisms. These hormones seem to modulate blood pressure (Reckelhoff, 2001). However, while the activation of estrogen receptors is associated with the reduction or attenuation of blood pressure, the action of male sex hormones leads to an elevation in blood pressure.

4. Sex Hormones and Hypertension

Sex hormones regulate a wide range of cellular events, as BP, an important factor in the development of hypertension and coronary artery disease, some of the most common cardiovascular diseases in the industrialized world (Orshal and Khalil, 2004). The sexual dimorphism may partly explain the differences observed in BP between men and women, which exhibit lower blood pressure levels over much of their life span compared with their age-matched counterparts (Maric-Bilkan and Manigrasso, 2012; Wang et al 2012). The high levels of endogenous estrogens in premenopausal women have been associated with lower risk for a number of diseases, such as hypertension, diabetes mellitus, obesity, vascular disease, and stroke compared with age-matched men (Barton et al. 2011, Wang et al. 2012). In addition, data from the National Health and Nutrition Examination Survey (NHANES) indicate that age-standardized hypertension prevalence rates are increasing in general, and there is no subgroup in which they are declining and among each race/ethnic this trends are more favorable in men than in women. Moreover, more recently, obesity or overweight have been increasing more in men than in women.

On the other hand, estrogen has shown protective effects on vascular function and heart failure that could have been implicated in the prevention of arterial hypertension (Knowlton and Lee, 2012; Maric-Bilkan and Manigrasso, 2012). However, this clear female benefit no longer exists after menopause, showing again the influence of sex hormones in the pathophysiology of cardiovascular disease.

4.1. Sex Hormones and Vascular Function

Numerous vascular effects of include modulation of vascular function and inflammatory response as well as metabolic and hemodynamic effects are attributed to female sex hormones. The vascular protection conferred by estrogen may be mediated indirectly by its influence on the metabolism of lipoproteins or by a direct action on the modulation of molecular pathways in the vessel wall, and more specifically on endothelial cells (Hermenegildo et al., 2002).

Many studies have disclosed that arterial relaxation mediated by estrogen could result from endothelial cell activation, which releases nitric oxide (NO) and leads to cGMP pathway activation in vascular smooth muscle cells (VSMC) that could activate calcium-activated potassium channels. However, this pathway is probably not the main route through which E2 elicits vasorelaxation, because it has been demonstrated several times that E2 can relax endothelium denuded arteries. With the use of pharmacological levels of E2, vascular relaxation in the absence of endothelium was correlated with decreased Ca^{2+} influx, increased K^+ efflux, and intracellular cAMP elevation in VSMC.

Estrogen also has a modulating effect on constrictive factors and positively up regulates the production of endothelium-derived relaxing factors such as PGI_2 and the endothelium-derived hyperpolarizing factors (EDHF) (Santos et al., 2010), both of which are important mediators of vascular relaxation in resistance sized arteries (figure 3).

In addition, estrogen increases NO bioavailability by mechanisms that either directly increase NO generation or decrease superoxide anion (O^{-2}) concentration, there by attenuating O^{2-} mediated NO inactivation. Estrogens such as 17β-estradiol, estrone, and estriol have been described to act as reactive oxygen species (ROS) scavengers by virtue of the hydrogen-donating capacity of their phenolic molecular structure.

The peripheral actions of estrogen could reduce development of hypertension through up-regulation of endothelium-derived vasodilator factors with simultaneous down-regulation of vasoconstrictor factors, such as endothelin-1 (Barber et al., 1996; Barber and Miller, 1998; Best et al., 1998; Dubey et al., 2001), inhibition of the renin-angiotensin system by reducing transcription of angiotensin-converting enzyme in endothelial cells (Brosnihan et al., 1994; Gallagher et al., 1999), and down-regulation of angiotensin 1 receptors (Nickenig et al., 1998).

Depletion of estrogen with a concomitant increase in androgens would, therefore, reduce local inhibitory signals while increasing pro contractile signals at the vascular wall, leading to increased peripheral resistance and blood pressure in the absence of concomitant decreases in sympathetic tone.

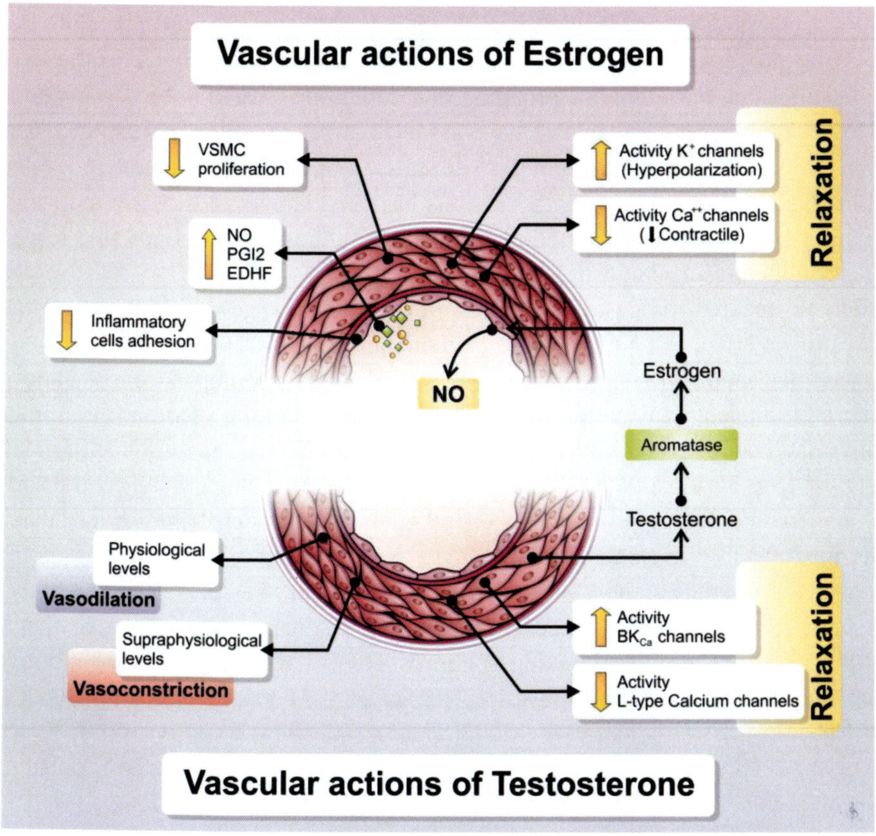

Figure 3. Vascular actions of estrogen and testosterone.

In addition to these direct effects on the vascular wall, in general, withdrawal of estrogen increases sympathetic tone as measured by increases in peripheral sympathetic neuronal activity and circulating levels of norepinephrine resulting in increased blood pressure, especially in the presence of a stressor (Saab et al., 1989; Owens et al., 1993; Vongpatanasin et al., 2001; Liu et al., 2003; Wyss and Carlson, 2003; Fernander et al., 2004). Furthermore, estrogen when injected directly into the brain, increases or decreases sympathetic tone depends upon the specific nuclei that are stimulated (Saleh and Connell, 2007) in this organ, ER seems to be localized in cardiovascular centers with inhibitory neurons (Blurton-Jones and Tuszynski, 2002). Thus, estrogen depletion would be associated with withdrawal of inhibitory tone such as that imparted by the parasympathetic system, thereby increasing peripheral resistance and lowering heart rate variability. Decreased heart rate variability was observed in women after oophorectomy compared with age-matched women who underwent hysterectomy with conservation of the ovaries. Heart rate variability was restored in the oophorectomized women after 3 months of estrogen therapy, although the type of estrogen therapy was not identified in this study (Mercuro et al., 2000).

Genetic variability in estrogen receptors and the ability to metabolize estrogen may be critical factors that could help to differentiate central autonomic effects of estrogen from those responses occurring at the level of the blood vessel wall in the systemic circulation.

The effects of both progesterone and its synthetic analogs (progestins) on the cardiovascular system in hormone replacement therapies are still controversial, which negatively seem to be involved in regulating numerous factors that influence the atherosclerotic process; affects circulating levels of various lipids, because the expression clotting factors, and thrombolytic proteins, and inhibiting vasodilation (Nakamura et al., 2005). However, experimental studies have associated these vascular effects to a dependent interaction progestogen type that binds to receptor. For example, natural progesterone in cultured human umbilical vein endothelial cells has been shown to increase the synthesis of NO, protein expression of eNOS, and activity eNOS, although it was not able to potentiate these effects in the presence of estrogen.

In addition, medroxyprogesterone acetate beyond not change any of these parameters, it inhibited estrogen effects on NO synthesis (Simoncini et al., 2004).

The vascular action of testosterone (Tes), in turn, seems to depend on its concentration (figure 3). The simplest explanation of this discrepancy is that the vasorelaxation induced by lower physiological concentrations of Tes appears to be, at least in part, endothelium dependent, whereas vasorelaxation induced by higher pharmacological concentrations of Tes in many *in vitro* studies appears to be endothelium independent (Perusquía at al., 2007; Rowell et al., 2009; Tep-areenan et al., 2002).

Although some studies show an action of endothelium, Tes acts predominantly on the vascular smooth muscle (VSM). Indeed, a variety of studies has demonstrated that the key mechanism underlying the vasorelaxing action of Tes is associated with the modulation of VSM cell membrane ion channel function, particularly *1)* inactivation of L-type voltage-operated Ca^{2+} channels (English et al., 2002; Hall et al., 2006) *2)* activation of K^+ channels (Cairraö et al., 2008; Seyrek et al., 2007), particularly the voltage-operated K^+ channel (Kv) and/or the large-conductance Ca^{2+}-activated K^+ channel (BK_{Ca}).

Moreover, Tes may also cause vasorelaxation by modulating intracellular signal transduction pathways such as increasing the levels of cGMP (Deenadayalu et al., 2001) and cAMP (Montaño , et al., 2008), which may indeed evoke vasorelaxation. In VSM cells, Tes stimulates NO production (via neuronal NOS), which in turn evokes the formation of cGMP (via guanylyl cyclase) to induce vasorelaxation (Deenadayalu et al., 2001). It has been reported that Tes increases cGMP accumulation and stimulates BK_{Ca} channel activity at micromolar concentrations (10–50 μM) in porcine coronary artery and at nanomolar concentrations (100 nM) in rat mesenteric myocytes to induce vasorelaxation (Deenadayalu et al., 2001). Second, the modulation of intracellular cAMP by Tes may occur via the sex hormone-binding globulin-Tes complex and may be biologically active via its binding to cell-surface sex hormone-binding globulin receptors that evoke an increase in intracellular cAMP. Thus Tes (120 nM) stimulates cAMP production in single rat aortic myocytes (Montaño , et al., 2008); then, the activation of cAMP induces the phosphorylation of protein kinase A and subsequently protein kinase A-mediated phosphorylation of either phospholamban (a protein that inhibits the sarcoplasmic reticulum ATPase Ca^{2+} pump), phospholipase C (enzyme responsible for inositol 1,4,5-trisphosphate production), or inositol 1,4,5-trisphosphate receptor, all of which are putative mechanisms of cAMP action.

4.2. Sex Hormones and Cardiac Function

It has been shown that testosterone has effects on cardiac muscle. It should be noted that cardiac muscle had androgen receptors (Kimura et al., 1993). In experimental myocardial infarction (left coronary artery ligation) in rats and mice, testosterone treatment caused maladaptive myocardial hypertrophy, with an increase in the beta / alpha-MHC-ratio and in IGF-1 expression (Nahrendorf et al., 2003; Frantz et al., 2007). There are some mechanism which could involve testosterone in left ventricular remodeling. Testosterone can increase collagens synthesis *in vivo* (Falanga et al., 1998) and levels of matrix metalloproteinase-9 early after myocardial infarction (Cavasin et al., 2006).

Male steroid hormone induces dose-dependent apoptotic cell death in adult rat ventricular myocytes *in vitro* (55). In addition, Aging-associated morphological and functional changes of cardiac and vascular myocytes lead to cardiac and vascular hypertrophy, fibrosis, decreased regenerative capacity of cardiac stem cells/endothelial progenitor cells (EPCs), increased myocyte death due to necrosis and apoptosis (Ungvari et al., 2010; Shih et al., 2011). Moreover, studies have pointed that high levels of testosterone (endogenous or supplemental) enhance acute myocardial inflammation and early remodeling, which adversely affect myocardial healing and impair cardiac function in mice after MI (Cavasin, 2006).

Regarding the electrical activity of the heart both acute intravenous and chronic transdermal testosterone therapy delay the onset of exercise- induced S-T segment depression in men with chronic, stable angina (Rosano et al., 1999; English et al., 2000). The steroid also extends total exercise time before development of myocardial ischemia and shortens return of the S-T segment to the isoelectric line (Rosano et al., 1999).

4.3. Sex Hormones and Renal System

The potential role of E2 in regulating renal function is evident from the observation that the kidney expresses the classic ERα and ERβ. In human fetal kidneys, ERβ is the prominent renal ER expressed, whereas ERα is only marginally expressed (Brandenberger et al., 1997). The data are controversial concerning adult renal tissue. In the kidney, E2 suppresses collagen synthesis in the glomerular mesangial cells (GMCs) by modulating mitogen activated protein (MAP) kinase activity and the expression of the transcription factor AP-1 (Zdunek et al., 2001; Silbiger et al., 1999; Neugarten et al., 1999), suggesting that E2 may limit the progression of glomerulosclerosis. Increased generation and deposition of extracellular matrix proteins (EMP) is the initial step in the development of glomerular injury and progressive loss of renal function. Clinical observations also indicate that E2 is indirectly involved in GMC growth by modulating the synthesis of growth promoters and growth inhibitors (Zdunek et al., 2001; Silbiger et al., 1999). E2 inhibits collagen synthesis induced by angiotensin II (ANG II) and transforming growth factor-β (TGF-β), which are implicated in the pathophysiology of progressive renal injury in kidney disease models. Moreover, E2 antagonizes the effects of TGF-β (Neugarten et al., 2002; Zdunek et al., 2001), on collagen synthesis and inhibits proliferation in GMCs. Previous investigations have also demonstrated that E2 attenuates ANG II-induced MAP kinase activity in GMCs, thus avoiding the deleterious effects of this peptide on the kidney.

It is important to note that, although the renal vasculature of male rats is more sensitive to the vasoconstrictor effects of ANG II, it is also more dependent on the vasodilator effects of NO compared to females, as demonstrated by the higher ANG II-induced increases in renal perfusion pressure in males compared to females, which remains the same between genders after blockade of NOS (Wangensteen et al., 2004). Therefore, it is possible that, because the male kidneys are more dependent on NO, the reduction in NO production during the aging process may uncover the presence of more vasoconstrictors, such as ANG II, thereby accelerating the progression of renal disease.

Androgens seem to confer cardioprotection. On the other hand, androgens can increase blood pressure and induce renal dysfunction, which may adversely influence the cardiovascular system (Lopes, et al., 2012). For example, clinical studies show reduced levels of testosterone in diabetic patients (Ding et al., 2006), raising the possibility that the severity of renal disease in these patients is partially due to a decrease in testosterone levels. The proximal tubule contains an autonomous renin-angiotensin system that can synthesize and luminally secrete angiotensin II or its precursors (Braam et al., 1999)

Interesting, castration of male rats lowers renal angiotensinogen mRNA levels by 60% and renal angiotensinogen mRNA levels rise to normal in castrated male rats when given replacement testosterone (Ellison et al., 1989). In addition, castration of male mice lowers activity of the Na/H exchanger, a brush-border membrane transporter regulated by angiotensin II and subsequent testosterone replacement raises and normalizes Na/H activity levels (Mackovic et al., 1986).

There is no conclusive data on the action of testosterone on the kidneys. In other word, It is unknown whether renal dysfunction or renal protection by testosterone is associated with direct effects of testosterone on the renal cells, or indirect effects of the hormone (Lopes, 2012). However, because human renal proximal tubule and cortical collecting duct cells express enzymes involved in androgen synthesis (Quinkler et al., 2003) as well as androgen receptors (Kimura et al., 1993)and tempting to assume that testosterone can regulates renal function by direct mechanisms.

Moreover, there are observations in experimental models that testosterone replacement can increase BP by such mechanisms as: increased oxidative stress, enhancement of tubular sodium and water reabsorption, activation of the renal renin–angiotensin system and endothelin and reduced nitric oxide availability (Reckelhoff et al., 2005).

Androgens appear to play an important role in the pathogenesis of hypertension and in modulating sex-specific differences in hypertension. This hypothesis is supported by the finding that experimental models which mimic hypertension or treatment with the androgen receptor antagonist flutamide lower blood pressure and slows the progression of hypertensive organ damage to the kidney. Apart from, administration of testosterone to these experimental models resulted in increases in blood pressure and renal injury subsequently showed fast progression. This effect could be mediated directly via activation of the renin angiotensin system or via increased proximal tubular reabsorption (Reckelhoff et al., 1999; Reckelhoff and. Granger, 1999; Reckelhoff el al., 1998).

Testosterone also is known to be profibrotic since it stimulates extracellular matrix proteins deposition in glomerular mesangial cells, leading to mesangial expansion and renal dysfunction (Lombet el tal., 1989). Experimental studies show that male rat mesangial cells express higher baseline fibronectin mRNA levels than female rat mesangial cells. Furthermore this investigation also demonstrated that basal cytokines such as tumor necrosis factor-α (TNF-α) and interleukin-1β levels are higher in male mesangial cells compared to female mesangial cells, indicating proinflammatory and profibrotic actions of testosterone in the kidney. (Pawluczyk et al., 2009)

Androgens also have been shown to increase proapoptotic signaling (Metcalfe et al., 2008). Testosterone-induced apoptosis in proximal tubule cells involves the activation of inflammatory cytokines, such as c-Jun amino terminal kinase and can be blocked by the AR antagonist flutamide, which reduces c-Jun amino terminal kinase phosphorylation (Verzola et al., 2009). These findings indicate that testosterone may play a crucial role in the acceleration of the tubular apoptotic process and the progression of chronic kidney disease in males.

Although data on testosterone and androgens being deleterious or beneficial to the cardiovascular and renal systems are still very controversial, in general, experimental evidence indicates that testosterone is essential for the equilibrium in the actions of many endothelium-derived vasoactive agents as well as for the appropriate function of structural components of these systems (Lopes et al., 2012).

4.4. Sex Hormones and Other Systems

Despite the higher prevalence of idiopathic pulmonary hypertension (PH) in young women, female animal models with PH induced exhibit less severe PH than their male counterparts; A recent study (Umar et al., 2011) shown that estrogen exerts protective effects on the progression of PH and can reversed it by improving cardiac and pulmonary structure and function. The fact that postmenopausal women have an increased risk for the development of pulmonary hypertension, and that hormone replacement therapy may prevent the development of PH in these patients further supports the beneficial role of E2 in patients with PH (Beretta et al., 2006).

Experimental studies using a PH model have consistently demonstrated hat administration of E2 exerts protective effects on the progression of PH. In pulmonary artery endothelial cells, estrogen acutely stimulates NO and NO synthase (NOS) release, up-regulate PGI2 and attenuates hypoxia-induced pulmonary ET-1 gene expression in lung tissue of adult female rats (Yuan et al., 2012). Additionally, estrogen treatment also suppressed the up-regulation of lung IL-6 transcript and protein levels induced by PH and reversed the loss of vessels associated with PH in the lungs in both male and female rats (Umar et al., 2011).

Estrogen also can exert protective effects in portal hypertension gastropathy in an experimental model by reduction the activities of antioxidant enzymes as superoxide dismutase, catalase and glutathione peroxidase and reduction lipoperoxidation in stomach (Morgan-Martins, 2011).

The reasons for the sex differences in baroreflex sensitivity and whether it involves neural, hormonal, or developmental factors are not clear. Short-term castration attenuates the vagal component of baroreflex sensitivity in sexually mature male rats and it has been shown that testosterone replacement restores baroreflex-mediated bradycardia in short-term castrated rats (El-Mas et al., 2001).

The mechanism by which testosterone modulates baroreflex responsiveness is not clear. Notwithstanding, testosterone has been shown to interact with at least two central mechanisms that are involved in baroreflex regulation. A) testosterone facilitates glutamatergic neurotransmission in several central areas including the hypothalamus (Pouliot et al., 1996) and hippocampus (Diano et al., 1997). Notably, glutamate is an essential neurotransmitter in the central processing of baroreceptor information (Van Giersbergen et al., 1992). B) testosterone increases the central expression of vasopressin mRNA (Wang et al., 1995) which is known to enhance baroreflex function (Peuler et al., 1990).

Interestingly, androgen receptors have been characterized in brainstem areas that are involved in baroreflex integration. In situ hybridization studies have identified androgen receptor mRNA–containing neurons in the nucleus tractus solitarius (Simerly et al., 1990), the central site of termination of baroreceptor afferents conveying information from arterial baroreceptors. Androgen receptors have been also demonstrated in the nucleus ambiguous and the dorsal motor nucleus of the vagus (Sheridan and Weaker, 1982), brainstem areas that play a crucial role in the control of central vagal discharges (Ciriello and Calaresu, 1979). It is possible, therefore, that androgen may act in these brainstem vagal centers to modulate the cardiomotor vagal activity.

5. New Perspectives on the Treatment of Hypertension by Sex Hormones

The years proximate to the menopause are accompanied by a rise in blood pressure and an increasing prevalence of hypertension. This increase in blood pressure may partially explain the corresponding marked and progressive increased risk of cardiovascular events observed in postmenopausal women (Preston et al., 2009). Among the known cardiovascular risk factors, the incidence of both dyslipidemia and hypertension stand. Lipid profile changes toward an atherogenic profile are observed in women after menopause, with an increase in low-density lipoprotein [LDL] cholesterol and a decrease in HDL cholesterol. The prevention of cardiovascular disease and its management in postmenopausal women is, therefore, a major health issue (Gompel et al., 2011).

Hormone therapy (HT) in postmenopausal women has been thought to provide an efficient protection against the progression of arterial disease by restoring the deficient estrogen (Gompel et al., 2011). Observational studies show that postmenopausal women who receive hormone replacement therapy (HRT) have a lower rate of CVD and cardiac death than those not receiving HRT (Yang et al., 2011). Nevertheless, these studies contrast with the large prospective clinical trials, Heart and Estrogen/Progestin Replacement Study (HERS I and II) and Women's Health Initiative (WHI), which failed to show reduced cardiovascular events in postmenopausal women on HRT (Rossouwetal, 2002; Yang et al., 2011). In fact, these trials suggested that HRT was associated with increased risk and events to the cardiovascular system, as stroke, venous thromboembolic disease and deep vein thrombosis (Sare et al., 2008).

The reasons for this paradoxical characterization of HRT have been extensively discussed. Many potential factors may contribute to the adverse outcome, among them the age of patients, preexisting CVD and/or risk, when HRT was initiated, the type of HRT given (conjugated equine estrogen with progestin), dosage, and the thromboembolic properties of estrogen and progestin (Yang et al., 2011).

In fact, in most observational studies, women started HRT around the time of menopause (which occurs on average at 51 years), whereas in others the average age of women entering in clinical trials, as WHI, was 65 years and older, which results in a study population with some degree of aging associated vascular damage. In addition, participants had been estrogen deficient for an average of 10 years before starting HRT, a relatively late start that could modify the status of ERs and molecular signaling so as to attenuate the benefits of estrogen.

Despite of the controversy about the benefits of estrogen replacement therapy in postmenopausal women, much recent interest has focused on whether replacing ovarian hormones can change the pattern of blood pressure alterations and affect the natural history of hypertension in postmenopausal women. There is experimental evidence that HRT reduces the incidence of hypertension in postmenopausal women, by exerting a direct effect on blood vessels through modulation of endogenous vasoconstrictors and vasodilators (Franco et al., 2002).

The cardiovascular benefits of estrogen have been attributed to its modulatory effects on NO generation by NOS isoforms (Xing et al., 2009). Estrogen deficiency, induced by ovariectomy, further increased aging-associated vasoconstriction and impaired NO signaling (Stice et al., 2009; Novella et al., 2010). Estrogen replacement also improved flow-induced vasodilation in coronary arterioles of aged and ovariectomized rats and restored eNOS phosphorylation (Ser1176), suggesting a positive regulation of estrogen on eNOS activity in old females (LeBlanc et al., 2009). In addition, untreated postmenopausal women have reduced circulating levels of NO (diminished nitrite/nitrate levels), raised endothelin-1 levels and impaired endothelial function in comparison with postmenopausal women treated with HRT (Franco et al., 2002).

Prospective studies in humans have shown variable effects of HRT on blood pressure in normotensive and hypertensive postmenopausal women (Franco et al., 2002). The Postmenopausal Estrogen/Progestin Interventions trial found no significant difference in blood pressure as a function of HRT (conjugated equine estrogen ± native or synthetic progestin) use. On the other hand, the WHI found an increase in blood pressure with hormone replacement therapy (conjugated equine estrogen and medroxyprogesterone acetate). Furthermore, several recent clinical trials have uniformly demonstrated that HRT in combination with drospirenone/17β-estradiol lowers blood pressure in hypertensive postmenopausal women and has an additive lowering effect on blood pressure when administered in combination with existing antihypertensive therapy with angiotensin converting enzyme (ACE) inhibitors, angiotensin receptor antagonists and hydrochlorothiazide (Preston et al., 2009; Franco et al., 2002).

Currently, data concerning the influence of HRT on blood pressure in postmenopausal women are inconclusive because of the limitations of published studies, as discussed previously.

5.1. Hormone Replacement Therapy Alternative - SERMs (Selective Estrogen Receptor Modulators Selective)

SERMs are nonsteroidal molecules with tissue-specific estrogen agonist and antagonist effects. These compounds interact with the estrogen receptor at the ligand-binding domain and differentially recruit coactivators or co-repressors to produce their effects (Nilsson et al., 2005). The SERMs chosen for this study are the most widely prescribed, tamoxifen (TAM) and raloxifene (RAL). TAM is an estrogen antagonist in the breast, but an agonist in the endometrium (Osborne, 1998), and is used for the treatment of estrogen-sensitive breast cancer. RAL is an estrogen antagonist in the breast and uterus, but an estrogen agonist in the bone (Sato et al., 1996), and is widely used for the prevention and treatment of osteoporosis (Osborne, 1998). Evidence has shown that RAL, like estrogen, induces endothelium-dependent acute vasodilation (Figtree et al., 1999; Kim et al., 1999) and directly activates nitric oxide synthesis in endothelial cells, resulting in dilation of blood vessels.

It is well known that the physiological effects of estrogen on gene transcription are determined by a characteristic combination of an activator and co-repressor proteins co REs that interact with any given cell. Manipulation of these interactions may provide a rational basis for specific target cardiovascular system. Selective modulators of estrogen receptor (SERMs) are drugs that exhibit some specificity in their effects and tissue are suggested as drugs that may be used in postmenopausal women. A SERM raloxifene benzothiophene that estradiol is chemically distinct, is approved for the treatment and prevention of osteoporosis in postmenopausal women. Raloxifene has properties similar to estrogen on the cardiovascular system, such as reduction of the concentrations of serum cholesterol and LDL improve endothelial function, although it is antagonistic to the proliferative effects of estrogen on the uterus and breast. These properties of raloxifene provided the basis for the RUTH (Raloxifene Use for The Heart) randomized, controlled trial that studied its ability to decrease fatal myocardial infarction, fatal coronary disease and hospitalization for acute coronary syndrome. The RUTH trial commenced in 2001, with an average 5-year follow-up, and included 10,000 postmenopausal women > 55 years of age, and the study reported a reduced risk of invasive breast cancer, but a no effect of raloxifene on primary coronary events. Moreover, there was an increased risk of venous thromboembolism and fatal stroke. Thus further studies are needed to investigate its use in hormone therapy.

Another SERMs is tamoxifen is a non-steroidal, triphenylethylene derivative that is widely used and highly effective as adjuvant therapy for the management of breast cancer patients with estrogen receptor (ER) positive tumors. Originally developed in the 1960s as a contraceptive agent, tamoxifen was later found to stimulate ovulation, as well as inhibit the formation of mammary tumors in rats exposed to carcinogens. While tamoxifen itself is a poor ER ligand, its metabolite 4-hydroxytamoxifen is a potent antagonist with high affinity for the ER. Tamoxifen and/or its metabolites exert anti-estrogenic effects in breast tissue, estrogenic effects on bone (increased density) and plasma cholesterol (decreased levels), and mixed effects in the uterus. In addition to the beneficial effects of tamoxifen, its complex, tissue specific action can also result in adverse effects in women. Peri-menopausal symptoms of hot flushes and night sweats are frequently reported side effects in both pre- and post-menopausal women on tamoxifen therapy. In pre-menopausal women, tamoxifen has also been reported to cause oligomenorrhea or amenorrhea with a return to normal menses after discontinuing tamoxifen. Yet, the greatest concern has been focused on the effects of tamoxifen in the uterus. Tamoxifen treatment increases the relative risk for endometrial cancer and may increase the incidence of endometriosis and uterine mesenchymal (*i.e.* myometrial) tumors.

Tamoxifen could also alter vascular reactivity, including antagonism of several ion channels and calmodulin, and inhibition of myosin light chain kinase, are consistent with studies speculating that several potentially important tamoxifen actions are ER-independent. Clinical observations have shown that treatment with tamoxifen reduces the incidence of ischemic heart disease and coronary atherosclerosis. Other studies have also reported decreases in total serum cholesterol and HDL cholesterol with tamoxifen treatment. Additionally, in experimental studies, tamoxifen exerted effects similar to those of estrogen on vascular relaxation due to several mechanisms, including antagonism of various ion channels.

Conclusion

In this chapter we tried to provide a literature update on the role of endogenous sex steroids on cardiovascular disease and this implication in hypertension. The sexual hormones are able to prevent endothelial injury, with one exhibiting its own mechanism with distinct features, however clinical studies investigating associations between endogenous estrogen or androgen and vascular alterations in men and women in the pre- and postmenopausal period show rather inconsistent results. Both the male sex hormones and the female can act through genomic and non-genomic mechanisms and appear to modulate blood pressure. However, while the activation of estrogen receptors is associated with the reduction or attenuation of blood pressure, the action of male sex hormones leads to bidirectional effect on blood pressure that to depend on its concentration. The knowledge of the actions of sex hormones in hypertension could contribute to the development of more appropriate therapies to control blood pressure in postmenopausal women.

Acknowledgments

The Fabricio Bragança da Silva from the Postgraduate Program in Physiological Sciences, Federal University of Espírito Santo for creating the illustration made for this chapter.

References

Arias-Loza, P. A., Hu, K., Dienesch, C., Mehlich, A. M., König, S., Jazbutyte, V., Neyses. L., Hegele-Hartung, C., Fritzemeier, K. H., and Pelzer, T. 2007. Both Estrogen Receptor Subtypes, β and α, Attenuate Cardiovascular Remodeling in Treated Rats − Aldosterone Salt. *Hypertension*. 50, 432-43.

Barton, M., Meyer, M. R. and Prossnitz, E. R. 2011. Estrogen-Independent Activation of Estrogen Receptors. *Hypertension*, 57, 1056-1057.

Bhasin, S. and Jasuja, R. 2009. Selective androgen receptor modulators as function promoting therapies. *Curr. Opin. Clin. Nutr. Metab. Care* 12, 232-240.

Bookout, A. L., Jeong, Y., Downes, M., Yu, R. T., Evans, R. M., and Mangelsdorf, D. J. 2006. Anatomical profiling of nuclear receptor expression reveals a hierarchical transcriptional network. *Cell*. 125, 789–799.

Braam, B., Mitchell, K. D., Fox, J., and Navar, L. G. 1993. Proximal tubular secretion of angiotensin II in rats. *Am. J. Physiol. Renal. Fluid Electrolyte. Physiol*. 264, F891–F898.

Brandenberger, A. W., Tee, M. K., Lee, J. Y., Chao, V., and Jaffe, R. B. 1997. Tissue distribution of estrogen receptors alpha (ER-alpha) and beta (ER-beta) mRNA in the midgestational human fetus. *J. Clin. Endocrinol. Metab*. 82, 3509-3512.

Burger, N. Z., Kuzina, O. Y., Osol, G., and Gokina, N. I. 2009. Estrogen replacement enhances EDHF-mediated vasodilation of mesenteric and uterine resistance arteries: role of endothelial cell Ca^{2+} *Am. J. Physiol. Endocrinol. Metab*. 296,E503-E512.

Busse, R., Edwards, G., Feletou, M., Fleming, I., Vanhoutte, P. M., and Weston, A. H. 2002. EDHF: bringing the concepts together. *Trends Pharmacol. Sci.* 23, 374–380.

Cairraö, E., Alvarez, E., Santos-Silva, A. J., and Verde, I. 2008. Potassium channels are involved in testosterone-induced vasorelaxation of human umbilical artery. *Naunyn Schmiedebergs Arch. Pharmacol.* 376, 375–383.

Cavasin, M. A., Tao, Z. Y. and Yu, X. P. 2006. Testosterone enhances early cardiac remodeling after myocardial infarction, causing rupture and degrading cardiac function. *Am. J. Physiol. Heart Circ. Physiol.* 290, H2043-2050.

Ciriello, J. and Calaresu, F. R. 1979. Separate medullary pathways mediating reflex vagal bradycardia to stimulation of buffer nerves in the cat. *J. Auton. Nerv. Syst.* 1, 13–32.

Conneely, O. M., Mulac-Jericevic, B., DeMayo, F., Lydon, J. P., and O'Malley, B. M. 2002. Reproductive Functions of Progesterone Receptors. *Recent Prog. Horm. Res.* 57, 339-55.

Cosman, F. and Lindsay, R. 1999. Selective Estrogen Receptor Modulators: Clinical Spectrum. *Endocr. Rev.* 20 (3), 418-34.

Cutini, P. H., Campelo, A. E., Agriello, E., Sandoval, M. J., Rauschemberger, M. B., and Massheimer, V. L. 2012. The role of sex steroids on cellular events involved in vascular disease. *J. Steroid Biochem. and Mol. Biol.* 132, 322–330.

Deenadayalu, V. P., White, R. E., Stallone, J. N., Gao, X., and Garcia, A. J. 2001. Testosterone relaxes coronary arteries by opening the large-conductance, calcium activated potassium channel. *Am. J. Physiol. Heart Circ. Physiol.* 281, H1720–H1727.

Dessy, C., Feron, O. and Balligand, J. L. 2010. The regulation of endothelial nitric oxide synthase by caveolin: a paradigm validated in vivo and share by the 'endothelium-derived hyperpolarizing factor'. *Pflügers Arch. Eur. J. Physiol.* 459, 817–827.

Dhote, V. V. and Balaraman, R. 2007. Gender specific effect of progesterone on myocardial ischemia/reperfusion injury in rats. *Life Sciences*. 81, 188–197.

Diamond, J. R. and Karnovsky, M. J. 1988. Focal and segmental glomerulosclerosis: analogies to atherosclerosis. *Kidney Int*. 33, 917-924.

Diano, S., Naftolin, F. and Horvath, T. H. 1997. Gonadal steroids target AMPA glutamate receptor-containing neurons in the rat hypothalamus, septum and amygdala: a morphological and biochemical study. *Endocrinology* 138,778–89.

Ding, E. L., Song, Y., Malik, V. S., and Liu, S. 2006. Sex differences of endogenous sex hormones and risk of type 2 diabetes: a systematic review and meta-analysis. *JAMA* 295, 1288–1299.

Donaldson, C., Eder, S., Baker, C., Aronovitz, M. J., Weiss, A. D., Hall-Porter, M., Wang, F., Ackerman, A., Karas, R. H., Molkentin, J. D., and Pattern, R. D. 2009. Estrogen attenuates left ventricular and cardiomyocyte hypertrophy by an estrogen receptor-dependent pathway that increases calcineurin degradation. *Circ. Res.* 104, 265–275.

Downs, J. L. and Wise, P. M. 2009.The role of the brain in female reproductive aging. *Mol. Cell. Endocrinol.* 299, 32–38.

Dubey, R. K. and Jackson, E. K. 2001. Estrogen-induced cardio renal pro- tection: potential cellular, biochemical, and molecular mechanisms. *Am. J. Physiol. Renal. Physiol.* 280, F365– F388.

Dusting, G. J., Moncada, S. and Vane, J. R. 1977. Prostacyclin (PGX) is the endogenous metabolite responsible for relaxation of coronary arteries induced by arachindonic acid. *Prostaglandins* 13, 3–15.

Dutertre, M. and Smith, C. L. 2000. Molecular Mechanisms of Selective Estrogen Receptor Modulator (SERM) Action. *Pharmacol. Experimental Therapeutics* 295 (2), 431-437.

Ellison, K. E., Ingelfinger, J. R., Pivor, M., and Dzau, V. J. 1989. Androgen regulation of rat renal angiotensinogen messenger RNA expression. *J. Clin. Invest.* 83, 1941–1945.

El-Mas, M. M., Afify, E. A., Mohy El-Din, M. M., Omar, A. G., and Sharabi, F. M. 2001. Testosterone facilitates the baroreceptor control of reflex bradycardia: role of cardiac sympathetic and parasympathetic components. *J. Cardiovasc. Pharmacol.* 38, 754-763.

English, K. M., Jones, R. D., Jones, T. H., Morice, A. H., and Channer, K. S. 2002. Testosterone acts as a coronary vasodilator by a calcium antagonistic action. *J. Endocrinol. Invest.* 25, 455–458.

English, K. M., Steeds, R. P., Jones, T. H., Diver, M. J., and Channer, K. S. 2000. Low-dose transdermal testosterone therapy improves angina threshold in men with chronic stable angina. *Circulation* 102, 1906-11.

Falanga, V., Greenberg, S. A., Zhou, L., Ochoa, S. M., Roberts, A. B., Falabella, A., and Yamaguchi, Y. 1998. Stimulation of collagen syntheses by the anabolic steroid stanozolol. *J. Invest. Dermatol.* 111, 1193-1197.

Figtree, G. A., Lu, Y., Webb, C. M., and Collins, P. 1999. Raloxifene acutely relaxes rabbit coronary arteries by an estrogen receptor-dependent and nitric oxide-dependent mechanism. *Circulation* 100, 1095–1101.

Fleming, I. 2000. Cytochrome P450 2C is an EDHF synthase in coronary arteries. *Trends Cardiovasc. Med.* 10, 166–170.

Fleming, I. 2010. Molecular mechanisms underlying the activation of eNOS. *Pflügers Arch. Eur. J. Physiol.* 459, 793–806.

Fliegner, D., Schubert, C., Penkalla, A., Witt, H., Kararigas, G., Dworatzek, E., Staub, E., Martus, P., Ruiz Noppinger P., Kintscher U, Gustafsson, J. A., and Regitz-Zagrosek V. 2010. Female sex and estrogen receptor-β attenuate cardiac remodeling and apoptosis in pressure overload. *Am. J. Physiol. Regul. Integr. Comp. Physiol.* 298, 1597–1606.

Franco, V. and Oparil, S. 2002. Hormone replacement therapy and hypertension. *Curr. Opin. Nephrol. Hypertens.* 11, 229-235.

Frantz, S., Hu, K., Widder, J., Weckler, B., Scheuermann, H., Bauersachs, J., Ertl, G., Callies, F., and Allolio, B. 2007. Detrimental effects of testosterone on post-myocardial infarction remodelling in female rats. *J. Physiol. Pharmacol.* 58, 717–772.

Garefalakis, M. and Hickey, M. 2008. Role of androgens, progestins and tibolone in the treatment of menopausal symptoms: a review of the clinical evidence. *Clin. Interv. in Aging* 3(1), 1–8.

Gava, A. L., Freitas, F. P. S., Meyrelles, S. S., Silva, I. V., and Graceli, J. B. 2011. Gender-dependent effects of aging on the kidney. *Braz. J. Med. Biol. Res.* 44(9), 905-913.

Geraldes, P., Sirois, M. G., Bernatchez, P. N., and Tanguay, J. F. 2002. Estrogen regulation of endothelial and smooth muscle cell migration and proliferation: role of p38 and p42/44 mitogen-activated protein kinase. *Arterioscler. Thromb. Vasc. Biol.* 22, 1585–1590.

Giguère, V. 2008. Transcriptional control of energy homeostasis by the estrogen-related receptors. *Endocr. Rev.* 124, 789–799.

Gilglioni, E. H., Campos, L. B., Oliveira, M. C., Garcia, R. F., Ambiel, C. R., Buzzo, A. J. R., Ishii-Iwamoto, E. L., and Salgueiro-Pagadigorria, C. L. 2012. Beneficial Effects of Tibolone on Blood Pressure and Liver Redox Status in Ovariectomized Rats With

Renovascular Hypertension. *J. Gerontol. A Biol. Sci. Med. Oct.* 22. [Epub. ahead of print].

Gompel, A., Boutouyrie P., Joannides, R., Christin-Maitre, S., Kearny-Schwartz, A., Kunz, K., Laurent, S., Boivin, J. M., Pannier, B., Pornel, B., Thuillez, C., Van Bortel, L., Zannad, F., Pithoois-Merli, I., Jaillon, P., and Simon, T. 2011. Association of menopause and hormone replacement therapy with large artery remodeling. *Fertil. and Steril.* 96 (6), 1445-50.

Hall, J., Jones, R. D., Jones, T. H., Channer, K. S., and Peers, C. 2006. Selective inhibition of L-type Ca2_ channels in A7r5 cells by physiological levels of testosterone. *Endocrinology* 147, 2675–2680.

Halliwell, B. and Grootveld, M. 1987. The measurement of free radical reactions in humans. Some thoughts for future experimentation. *FEBS Lett.* 213, 9–14.

Hamilton, K. L., Lin, L., Wang, Y., and Knowlton, A. A. 2007. Effect of ovariectomy on cardiac gene expression: inflammation and changes in SOCS genes expression. *Physiol. Genomics*. 32, 254–263.

Kang, L., Zhang, X., Xie, Y., Tu, Y.,Wang, D., Liu, Z., and Wang, Z.Y. 2010. Involvement of estrogen receptor variant ER-α36, Not GPR30, in nongenomic signaling. *Mol. Endocrinol*. 24, 709–721.

Karteris, E., Zervou, S., Pang, Y., Dong, J., Hillhouse, E. W., Randeva, H. S., and Thomas, P. 2006. Progesterone signaling in human myometrium through two novel membrane G protein-coupled receptors: potential role in functional progesterone withdrawal at term. *Mol. Endocrinol*. 20, 1519-1534.

Kim, H. P., Lee, J. Y., Jeong, J. K., Bae, S. W., Lee, H. K., and Jo, I. 1999. Nongenomic stimulation of nitric oxide release by estrogen is mediated by estrogen receptor alpha localized in caveolae. *Biochem. Biophys. Res. Commun*. 263, 257–262.

Kim, N. N., Stankovic, M., Armagan, A., Cushman, T. T., Goldstein, I., and Traish, A. M. 2006. Effects of tamoxifen on vaginal blood flow and epithelial morphology in the rat. *BMC Women's Health* 13, 6-14.

Kimura, N., Mizokami, A., Oonuma, T., Sasano, H., and Nagura, H. 1993. Immunocytochemical localization of androgen receptor with polyclonal antibody in paraffin- embedded human tissues. *J. His- tochem.Cytoche.* 41, 671–678.

Kimura, N., Mizokami, A., Oonuma, T., Sasano, H., and Nagura, H. 1993. Immunocytochemical localization of androgen receptor with polyclonal antibody in paraffin-embedded human tissues. *J. Histochem. Cytochem*. 41, 671-678.

Knowlton, A. A. and Lee, A. R. 2012. Estrogen and the cardiovascular system. *Pharmacol. and Ther*. 135, 54–70.

Kublickiene, K. and Luksha, L. 2008. Gender and the endothelium. *Pharmacol. Report*. 60, 49-60.

LeBlanc, A. J., Reyes, R., Kang, L. S., Dailey, R. A., Stallone, J. N., Moningka, N. S., and Muller-Delp, J. M. 2009. Estrogen replacement restores flow-induced vasodilation in coronary arterioles of aged and ovariectomized rats. *Am. J. Physiol. Regul. Integr. Comp. Physiol.* 297, 1713-1723.

Leonhardt, S. A., Boonyaratanakornkit, V. and Edwards, D. P. 2003 Progesterone receptor transcription and non-transcription signaling mechanisms. *Steroids* 68, 761–770.

Lombet, J. R., Adler, S. G., Anderson, P. S., Nast, C. C., Olsen, D. R., and Glassock, R. J. 1989. Sex vulnerability in the subtotal nephrectomy model of glomerulosclerosis in the rat. *J. Lab. Clin. Med.* 114, 66-74.

Lopes, R. A. M., Neves, K. B., Carneiro, F. S., and Tostes, R. C. 2012. Testosterone and vascular function in aging. *Frontiers in physiol.* 3, 1-9.

Mackovic, M., Zimolo, Z., Burckhardt, G., and Sabolic, I. 1986. Isolation of renal brush-border membrane vesicles by a low-speed centrifugation: effect of sex hormones on Na_-H_ exchange in rat and mouse kidney. *Biochim. Biophys. Acta* 862, 141–152.

Maric-Bilkan, C. and Manigrasso, M. B. 2012 Differences in Hypertension: Contribution of the Renin–Angiotensin System. *Gend. Med.* 9(4), 287-91.

McCredie, R. J., McCrohon, J. A., Turner L., Griffiths, K. A., Handelsman, D. J., and Celermajer, D. S. 1998. Vascular reactivity is impaired in genetic females taking high-dose androgens. *J. Am. Coll. Cardiol.* 32, 1331–1335.

Medeiros, A. N. S., Lamas, A. Z., Caliman, I. F., Dalpiaz, P. L., Firmes, L. B., Abreu, G. R., Moysés, M. R., Lemos, E. M., Reis, A. M., and Bissoli, N. S. 2012. Tibolone has anti-inflammatory effects in estrogen-deficient female rats on the natriuretic peptide system and TNF-alpha. *Regul. Pept.* 179(1-3), 55-60.

Metcalfe, P. D., Leslie, J. A., Campbell, M. T., Meldrum D. R., Hile, K. L., and Meldrum, K. K. 2008. Testosterone exacerbates obstructive renal injury by stimulating TNF-alpha production and increasing proapoptotic and profibrotic signaling. *Am. J. Physiol Endocrinol. Metab.* 294, E435-E443.

Miller, V. M. and Duckles, S. P. 2008. Vascular Actions of Estrogens: Functional Implications. *Pharmacol. Rev.* 60, 210–241.

Miller, V. M. 2010. Sex-based differences in vascular function. *Women's Health* 6(5), 737–752.

Mitchell, J. A., Ali, F., Bailey, L., Moreno, L., and Harrington, L. S. 2007. Role of NO and prostacyclin as vasoactive hormones released by the endothelium. *Exp. Physiol.* 3, 85–88.

Momoi, H., Ikomi, F. and Ohhashi, T. 2003. Estrogen-induced augmentation of endothelium-dependent nitric oxide mediated vasodilation in isolated rat cerebral small arteries. *Jpn. J. Physiol.* 53, 193–203.

Montaño, L. M., Calixto, E., Figueroa, A., Flores-Soto, E., Carbajal, V., and Perusquía, M. 2008. Relaxation of androgens on rat thoracic aorta: testosterone concentration dependent agonist/antagonist L-type Ca2_ channel activity, and 5beta-dihydrotestosterone restricted to L-type Ca2_ channel blockade. *Endocrinology* 149, 2517–2526.

Morgan-Martins, M. I., Jacques, S. I., Harrtmann, R. M., Marques, C. M., Marroni, C. A., and Marroni, N. P. 2011. Protection of Estrogen in Portal Hypertension Gastropathy – an experimental model. *Arq. Gastroenterol.* 48 (3), 211-216.

Muehlfelder, M., Arias-Loza, P. A., Fritzemeier, K. H., and Pelzer, T. 2012. Both estrogen receptor subtypes, ERa and ERb, prevent aldosterone-induced oxidative stress in VSMC via increased NADPH bioavailability. *Biochem. Biophys. Res. Commun.* 423, 850–856.

Nahrendorf, M., Frantz, S., Hu, K., von zur Mühlen, C., Tomaszewski, M., Scheuermann, H., Kaiser, R., Jazbutyte, V., Beer, S., Bauer, W., Neubauer, S., Ertl, G., Allolio, B., and Callies, F .2003. Effect of testosterone on post-myocardial infarction remodeling and function. *Cardiovasc. Res.* 57, 370–378.

Nakamura, Y., Suzuki, T., Inoue, P., Tazawaka, C., Ono, K., Moriya, T., Saito, H., Ishibashi, T., Takahashi, S., Yamada, S., and Sasano, H. 2005. Progesterone receptors subtypes in vascular smooth cells of human aorta. *Endocr. J.* 52 (2), 245-252.

Negro-Vilar, A. 1999. Selective androgen receptor modulators (SARMs): a novel approach to androgen therapy for the new millennium. *J. Clin. Endocrinol. Metab.* 84, 3459–3462.

Nettleship, J. E., Jones, R. D., Channer, K. S., and Jones, T. H. 2009. Testosterone and coronary artery disease. *Front Horm. Res.* 37, 91–107.

Neugarten, J., Kasiske, B., Silbiger, S. R., and Nyengaard, J. R. 2002. Effects of sex on renal structure. *Nephron* 90, 139-144.

Neugarten, J., Medve, I., Lei, J., and Silbiger, S. R. 1999. Estradiol suppresses mesangial cell type I collagen synthesis via activation activation of the MAP kinase cascade. *Am. J. Physiol.* 277, F875-F881.

Nilsson, S. and Koehler, K. F. 2005. Oestrogen receptors and selective oestrogen receptor modulators: molecular and cellular pharmacology. *Basic Clin. Pharmacol. Toxicol.* 96, 15–25.

Novella, S., Dantas, A. P., Segarra, G., Novensa, L., Heras, M., Hermenegildo, C., and Medina, P. 2011. Aging enhances contraction to thromboxane A(2) in aorta from female senescence-accelerated mice. *Age* (Dordr.) PMID: 22102320. [Epub. ahead of print].

Orshal, J. M. and Khalil, R. A. 2004. Gender, sex hormones, and vascular tone. *Am. J. Physiol. Regul. Integr. Comp. Physiol.* 286, R233–R249.

Osborne, C. K. 1998. Tamoxifen in the treatment of breast cancer. *N Engl. J. Med.* 339, 1609–1618.

Pare, G., Krust, A., Karas, R. H., Dupont, S., Aronovitz, M., Chambon, P., and Mendelsohn, M. E. 2002. Estrogen receptor-α mediates the protective effects of estrogen against vascular injury. *Circ. Res.* 90, 1087–1092.

Pathirana, I. N., Kawate, N., Büllesbach, E. E., Takahashi, M., Hatoya, S., Inaba, T., and Tamada, H. 2012. Insulin-like peptide 3 stimulates testosterone secretion in mouse Leydig cells via cAMP pathway Regul. *Pept.* 178, 102-6.

Pawluczyk, I. Z., Tan, E. K. and Harris, K. P. 2009. Rat mesangial cells exhibit sex-specific profibrotic and proinflammatory phenotypes. *Nephrol. Dial. Transplant.* 24, 1753-1758.

Pedram, A., Razandi, M., Lubahn, D., Liu, J., Vannan, M., and Levin, E. R. 2008. Estrogen inhibits cardiac hypertrophy: role of estrogen receptor-β to inhibit calcineurin. *Endocrinology.* 149, 3361–3369.

Perusquía, M., Navarrete, E., Gonzalez, L., and Villalón, C. M. 2007. The modulatory role of androgens and progestins in the induction of vasorelaxation in human umbilical artery. *Life Sci.* 81, 993–1002.

Peuler, J. D., Edwards, G. L., Schmid, P. G., and Johnson, A. K. 1990. Area postrema and differential reflex effects of vasopressin and phenylephrine in rats. *Am. J. Physiol.* 258, H1255–1259.

Pouliot, W. A., Handa, R. J. and Beck, S. G. 1996. Androgen modulates *N*-methyl-D-aspartate-mediated depolarization in CA1 hippocampal pyramidal cells. *Synapse* 23, 10 – 9.

Preston, R. A. 2009. Comparative effects of conventional vs. novel hormone replacement therapy on blood pressure in postmenopausal women. *Climacteric.* 12, 66–70.

Qiao, X., McConnell, K. R. and Khalil, R. A. 2008. Sex Steroids and Vascular Responses in Hypertension and Aging. *Gend. Med.* 5 Suppl. A:S46-64.

Quinkler, M., Bumke-Vogt, C., Meyer, B., Bahr, V., Oelkers, W., and Diederich, S. 2003. The human kidney is a progesterone-metabolizing and androgen-producing organ. *J. Clin. Endocrinol. Metab.* 88, 2803–2809.

Reckelhoff, J. F. and Granger, J. P. 1999. Role of androgens in mediating hypertension and renal injury. *Clin. Exp. Pharmacol. Physiol.* 26, 127–131

Reckelhoff, J. F. 2001. Gender differences in the regulation of blood pressure. *Hypertension* 37, 1199–1208.

Reckelhoff, J. F. 2001. Gender differences in the regulation of blood pressure. *Hypertension* 37, 1199–1208.

Reckelhoff, J. F., Yanes, L. L., Iliescu, R., Fortepiani, L. A., and Granger, J. P. 2005. Testosterone supplementation in aging men and women: possible impact on cardiovascular–renal disease. *Am. J. Physiol. Renal. Physiol.* 289, F941–F948.

Reckelhoff, J. F., Zhang, H. and Granger, J. P. 1998. Testosterone exacerbates hypertension and reduces pressure-natriuresis in male spontaneously hypertensive rats. *Hypertension* 31, 435–439

Reckelhoff, J. F., Zhang, H., Srivastava, K., and Granger, J. P. 1999. Gender differences in hypertension in spontaneously hypertensive rats: role of androgens and androgen receptor. *Hypertension* 34, 920–923

Rosano, G. M. C., Leonardo, F., Pagnotta, P., Pelliccia, F., Panina, G., Cerquetani, E., della Monica, P. L., Bonfigli, B., Volpe, M., and Chierchia, S. L. 1999. Acute anti-ischemic effect of testosterone in men with coronary artery disease. *Circulation* 99, 1666-70.

Rossouw, J. E., Prentice, R. L., Manson, J. E., Wu, L., Barad, D., Barnabei, V. M., Ko, M. Lacroix, A. Z., Margolis, K. L., Stefanick, M. L. 2007. Postmenopausal hormone therapy and risk of cardiovascular disease by age and years since menopause. *JAMA*. 297, 1465–1477.

Rowell, K. O., Hall, J., Pugh, P. J., Jones, T. H., Channer, K. S., and Jones, R. D. 2009. Testosterone acts as an efficacious vasodilator in isolated human pulmonary arteries and veins: evidence for a biphasic effect at physiological and supra-physiological concentrations. *J. Endocrinol. Invest.* 32, 718–723.

Rymer, J. 2002. Why tibolone is different? *Reviews in Gynaecological Practice* 2, 35–39.

Santos, R. L., Marin, E. B., Gonc¸alves, W. L. S., Bissoli, N. S., Abreu, G. R., and Moyses, M. R. 2010. Sex differences in the coronary vasodilation induced by 17 β-oestradiol in the isolated perfused heart from spontaneously hypertensive rats. *Acta Physiol.* 200, 203–210

Santos, R. L., Abreu, G. R., Bissoli, N. S., and Moysés, M. R. 2004. Endothelial mediators of 17ß-estradiol-induced coronary vasodilation in the isolated rat heart. *Braz. J. Med. Biol. Res.* 37, 569-575.

Sare G. M., Gray, L. J. and Philip, M. W. Bath. 2008. Association between hormone replacement therapy and subsequent arterial and venous vascular events: a meta-analysis. *Eur. Heart J.* 29, 2031–2041.

Sarkar, D. K., Chiappa, S. A., Fink, G., and Sherwood, N. M. 1976. Gonadotropin-releasing hormone surge in pro-oestrous rats. *Nature* 264 (5585), 461-3.

Sato, M., Rippy, M. K. and Bryant, H. U. 1996. Raloxifene, tamoxifen, nafoxidine, or estrogen effects on reproductive and nonreproductive tissues in ovariectomized rats. *FASEB J.* 10, 905–912.

Scarpin, K. M., Graham, J. D., Mote, P. A., and Clarke, C. L. 2009. Progesterone action in human tissues: regulation by progesterone receptor (PR) isoform expression, nuclear positioning and coregulator expression. *NURSA* 7, 01-13.

Schreiber, S. N., Knutti, D., Brogli, K., Uhlmann, T., and Kralli, A. 2003. The transcriptional coactivator PGC-1 regulates the expression and activity of the orphan nuclear receptor ERRα. *J. Biol. Chem.* 278, 9013–9018.

Seyrek, M., Yildiz, O., Ulusoy, H. B., and Yildirim, V. 2007. Testosterone relaxes isolated human radial artery by potassium channel opening action. *J. Pharm. Sci.* 103, 309–316.

Shaw, N. D., Srouji, S. S., Histed, S. N., and Hall, J. E. 2011.Differential effects of aging on estrogen negative and positive feedback. *Am. J. Physiol. Endocrinol. Metab.* 301, E351–E355.

Shaw, N. D., Srouji, S. S., Histed, S. N., McCurnin, K. E., and Hall, J. E. 2009. Aging attenuates the pituitary response to gonadotropin releasing hormone. *J. Clin. Endocrinol. Metab*. 94, 3259–3264.

Sheridan, P. J. and Weaker, F. J. 1982. Androgen receptor systems in the brain stem of the primate. *Brain Res.* 235, 225–32.

Shih, H., Lee, B., Lee, R. J., and Boyle, A. J. 2011. The aging heart and post- infarction left ventricular remodeling. *J. Am. Coll Cardiol*. 57, 9–17.

Shimokawa, H., Yasutake, H., Fujii, K., Owada, M. K., Nakaike, R., Fukumoto, Y., Takayanagi, T., Nagao, T., Egashira, K., Fujishima, M., and Takeshita, A. 1996. The importance of the hyperpolarizing mechanism increases as the vessel size decreases in endothelium-dependent relaxations in rat mesenteric circulation. *J. Cardiovasc. Pharmacol*. 28, 703–711.

Silbiger, S., Lei, J. and Neugarten, J. 1999. Estradiol suppresses type I collagen synthesis in mesangial cells via activation of activator protein-1. *Kidney Int*. 55, 1268-1276.

Simerly, R. B., Chang, C., Muramatsu, M., and Swanson, L. W. 1990. Distribution of androgen and estrogen receptor mRNA-containing cells in the rat brain: an in situ hybridization study. *J. Comp. Neurol*. 294, 76–95.

Simoncini, T. and Genazzani, A. R. 2000. Tibolone inhibits leukocyte adhesion molecule expression in human endothelial cells. *Mol. Cell. Endocrin.* 162, 87–94.

Simoncini, T., Mannella, P., Fornari, L., Caruso, A., Willis, M. Y., Garibalde, S., Baldacci, C., Genazzani, A. R. 2004. Differential Signal Transduction of Progesterone and Medroxyprogesterone Acetate in Human Endothelial Cells. *Endocrinology*, December 2004, 145 (12):5745–5756.

Souza, M. A. M., Souza, B. M. and Geber, S. 2012. Vascular resistance of central retinal and ophthalmic arteries in postmenopausal women after use of tibolone. Menopause: *The Journal of The North American Menopause Society* 19 (3), 328-331.

Stice, J. P., Elserich, J. P., Knowlton, A. A. 2009. Role of Aging Versus the Loss of Estrogens in the Reduction in Vascular Function in Female Rats. *Endocrinology,* 150 (1), 212–219.

Stice, J. P., Chen, L., Kim, S. C., Chen, L., Tran, A. L., Liu, T. T., and Knowlton, A. A. 2011. 17β-estradiol, aging, inflammation and the stress response in the female heart. *Endocrinology*. 152, 1589–1598.

Takahashi, K., Ohmichi, M., Yoshida, M., Hisamoto, K., Mabuchi, S., Arimoto-Ishida, E., Mori, A., Tsutsumi, S., Tasaka, K., Murata, Y., and Kurachi, H. 2003. Both estrogen and raloxifene cause G1 arrest of vascular smooth muscle cells. *J. Endocrinol.* 178, 319–329.

Tep-areenan, P., Kendall, D. A. and Randall, M. D. 2002. Testosterone-induced vasorelaxation in the rat mesenteric arterial bed is mediated predominantly via potassium channels. *Br. J. Pharmacol.* 135, 735–740.

Thomas, P., Pang, Y., Dong, J., Groenen, P., Kelder, J., de Vlieg,. J, Zhu Y., and Tubbs, C. 2007. Steroid and G protein binding characteristics of the seatrout and human progestin membrane receptor alpha subtypes and their evolutionary origins. *Endocrinology* 148, 705-718.

Traish, A. M., Guay, A., Feeley, R., and Saad, F. 2009. The dark side of testosterone deficiency: I. Metabolic syndrome and erectile dysfunction. *J. Androl.* 30, 10–22.

Umar, S., Iorga, A., Matori, H., Nadadur, R. G., Li, J., Maltase, F., Laarse, A., and Eghbali, M. 2011. Estrogen Rescues Preexistentig severe pulmonary hypertension in rats. *Am. J. Respir. Crit. Care Med.* 184, 715–723.

Ungvari, Z., Kaley, G., deCabo, R., Songtag, W. E., and Csiszar, A. 2010. Mechanisms of vascular aging: new perspectives. *J. Gerontol. A Biol. Sci. MedSci.* 65, 1028–1041.

Van Giersbergen, P. L. M., Palkovits, M. and De Jong, W. 1992. Involvement of neurotransmitters in the nucleus tractus solitari in cardiovascular regulation. *Physiol. Rev.* 72, 789–824.

Verzola, D., Illaggio, B., Procopio, V., Gandolfo, M. T., Gianiorio, F., Fama, A., Tosetti, F., Traverso, P., Deferrari, G., and Garibotto, G. (2009) Androgen-mediated apoptosis of kidney tubule cells: role of c-Jun amino terminal kinase. *Biochem. Biophys. Res. Commun.* 387, 531-536.

Wang, L., Szklo, M., Folsom, A. R., Cook, N. R., Gapstur, S. M., and Ouyang, P. 2012. Endogenous sex hormones, blood pressure change, and risk of hypertension in postmenopausal women: The Multi-Ethnic Study of Atherosclerosis. *Atherosclerosis.* 224, 228-234.

Wang, L., Szklo, M., Folsom, A. R., Cook, N. R., Gapstur, S. M., and Ouyang, P. 2012. Endogenous sex hormones, blood pressure change, and risk of hypertension in postmenopausal women: The Multi-Ethnic Study of Atherosclerosis. *Atherosclerosis* 224, 228-234.

Wang, Z. and De Vries, G. T. 1995. Androgen and estrogen effects on vasopressin messenger RNA expression in the medial amygdaloid nucleus in male and female rats. *J. Neuroendocrinol.* 7, 827–831.

Wangensteen, R., Moreno, J. M., Sainz, J., Rodriguez-Gomez, I., Chamorro, V., Luna, J. D., Osuna, A., and Vargas, F. 2004. Gender difference in the role of endothelium-derived relaxing factors modulating renal vascular reactivity. *Eur. J. Pharmacol.* 486, 281-288.

Weiss, J. M., Huang, W. Y., Rinaldi, S., Fears, T. R., Chatterjee, N., Hsing, A. W., Crawford, E. D., Andriole, G. L., Kaaks, R., and Hayes, R. B. 2008. Endogenous sex hormones and the risk of prostate cancer: a prospective study. *Int. J. Cancer* 122, 2345-50.

Wilson, C. M. and McPhaul, M. J. 1996. □ and β forms of the androgen receptor are expressed in a variety of human tissues. *Mol. Cell. Endcorinol.* 120, 51–57.

Wise, P. M. 1982. Alterations in proestrous LH, FSH, and prolactin surges in middle-aged rats. *Proc. Soc. Exp. Biol. Med.* 169, 348–354.

Wu, Q., Chambliss, K. L., Umetani, M., Mineo, C., and Shaul, P. W. 2011. Non-nuclear estrogen receptor signaling in the endothelium. *J. Biol. Chem.* 286, 14737–14743.

Xing, D., Nozell, S., Chen, Y. F., Hage, F., and Oparil, S. 2009. Estrogen and Mechanisms of Vascular Protection. *Arterioscler. Thromb. Vasc. Biol.* 29, 289–295.

Yang, X. P. and Reckelhoff, J. F. 2011. Estrogen, hormonal replacement therapy and cardiovascular disease. *Hypertension.* 20, 133–138.

Yu, X., Handong, M., Barman, S. A., Liu, A. T., Sellers, M., Stallone, J. N., Prossnitz, E. R., White, R. E., and Han, G. 2011. Activation of G protein-coupled estrogen receptor induces endothelium-independent relaxation of coronary artery smooth muscle. *Am. J. Physiol. Endocrinol. Metab.* 301, E882–E888.

Yuan, P., Wu, W. H., Gao, L., Zheng, Z. Q., Liu, D., Mei, H. Y., Zhang, Z. L., and Jing, Z. C. 2012. Oestradiol ameliorates monocrotaline pulmonary hypertension via NO, PGI_2 and ET-1 pathways. *Eur. Respir. J.* Aug. 30. [Epub. ahead of print].

Zaugg, M., Jamali, N. Z., Lucchinetti, E., Xu, W., Alam, M., Shafiq, A. S., and Siddiqui, M. A. Q. 200. Anabolic-androgenic steroids induce apoptotic cell death in adult rat ventricular myocytes. *J. cel. Physiol.* 18790-95

Zdunek, M., Silbiger, S., Lei, J., and Neugarten, J. 2001. Protein kinase CK2 mediates TGF-beta1-stimulated type IV collagen gene transcription and its reversal by estradiol. *Kidney Int.* 60, 2097-2108.

Zhu, Y., Bian, Z., Lu, P., Karas, R.H., BAo, L., Cox, D., Hodgin, J., Shaul, P. W., Thoren, P., Smithies, O., Gustafsson, J. A., and Mendelshon, M. E. 2002. Abnormal Vascular Function and Hypertension in Mice Deficient in Estrogen Receptor β. *Science* 295, 505-508.

Zhu, Y., Bond, J. and Thomas, P. 2003. Identification, classification, and partial characterization of genes in humans and other vertebrates homologous to a fish membrane progestin receptor. *Proc. Natl. Acad. Sci. US* 100, 2237-2242.

Zhu, Y., Rice, C. D., Pang, Y., Pace, M., and Thomas, P. 2003. Cloning, expression, and characterization of a membrane progestin receptor and evidence it is an intermediary in meiotic maturation of fish oocytes. *Proc. Natl. Acad. Sci. US* 100, 2231-2236.

Zhuang, L. Z., Adashi, E. Y. and Hsueh, A. J. W. 1982. Direct enhancement of gonadotropin-stimulated ovarian estrogen biosynthesis by estrogen and clomiphene citrate. *Endocrinology* 110(6), 2219-21.

In: Arterial Hypertension
Editors: Marten Vosler and Siemen Weber
ISBN: 978-1-62417-852-8
© 2013 Nova Science Publishers, Inc.

Chapter 5

Arterial Hypertension in Children and Adolescence: Risk Factors

Sônia Alves Gouvêa,[1,2]* Renata Viana Tiradentes,[2] Cíntia Helena Santuzzi,[2,3] Gláucia Rodrigues de Abreu[1,2] and Anabel Nunes Rodrigues[3]

[1]Department of Physiological Sciences,
Federal University of Espírito Santo, Vitória, Brazil
[2]Postgraduate Program in Physiological Sciences,
Federal University of Espírito Santo, Vitória, Brazil
[3]School of Medicine, University Center of Espírito Santo, Colatina, Brazil

Abstract

This chapter will explore the importance of investigating the hypertension in childhood and adolescence that may emerge in adult life and debate a prevalence, incidence and occurrence of hypertension in children and adolescents, addition to addressing the methods and instruments used to determine hypertension, risk factors, health promotion, education and treatment for hypertensive children and adolescents.

Studies have shown significant rates of hypertension in children and adolescents and considering necessary to check blood pressure in childhood, since the increase in the arterial BP in youth indicates a prediction of hypertension in adulthood.

Studies involving analysis of hypertension risk factors should always register the prevalence and their correlations in childhood, as an essential to identify a population at risk. Therefore, the early detection of risk factors in asymptomatic children may contribute to a decrease in the development of hypertension and prevention of possible co morbidities.

* Corresponding author: Sonia Alves Gouvêa, PhD. Departamento de Ciências Fisiológicas – Centro de Ciências da Saúde da Universidade Federal do Espírito Santo, Avenida Marechal Campos, 1456 – Maruípe, Vitória, Espírito Santo – Brasil. CEP 29040-577; Tel.: +55 27 3335-7473/ 97033975; Fax: + 55 27 3335-7330; E-mail: sagouvea@ppgcf.ufes.br or gouveasa@yahoo.com.br.

In view of the substantial tracking of hypertension risk factors from adolescents to adulthood, there is an urgent need to intervene early with efficacious strategies to identify and treat hypertensive children and adolescents. The traditional hypertensive risk factors, namely overweight/obesity and family history, including lifestyle (a bad diet, stress, and insufficient physical activity) appear to be important, accounting for the dramatic recent changes in prevalence and would be of public health concern.

Keywords: Hypertension, children, adolescents, blood pressure, risk, cardiovascular disease, prevention, lifestyle changes

1. Introduction

Childhood can be considered the period of structuring of life, where patterns such as diet and lifestyle are built and the adolescence is a particular stage in the lifespan that is characterized as being between childhood and adulthood (Kelishadi et al., 2002). While adolescents vary in their experiences world-wide and in their degree of independence, adult responsibility, and access to education, it is a common experience that they begin the tasks of establishing their own identity within the wider culture and society within which they live. Their emerging independence includes beginning to exercise their own choices of food, physical activity or inactivity, smoking behaviors, sexual experiences, and social relationships (Kilty and Prentice, 2012).

The theory that primary (or essential) hypertension has its origins in the young was proposed in the first report from the National Heart Lung and Blood Institute (NHLBI) on high blood pressure (BP) in children, published in 1977 (Redwine and Falkner, 2012; Blumenthal et al., 1977). Over subsequent years the theory on childhood origins of hypertension has been supported by a substantial body of epidemiologic data that link higher BP levels in childhood with early onset hypertension in adulthood (Falkner, 2012). Cohort studies that obtained repeated measures of BP from childhood into young adulthood describe tracking of BP, with higher BP levels in childhood corresponding with higher BP levels in young adulthood. The BP tracking phenomenon was confirmed by Chen and Wang (2008) in their meta-analysis on 50 published cohort studies, representing diverse populations. Their analysis demonstrated an overall average tracking coefficient of 0.38 for systolic BP, thus confirming the observation that higher BP levels in childhood are associated with higher BP levels in young adulthood.

Both epidemiologic and clinical data in adults link a BP level above 140/90 mmHg with a marked increase in risk for morbid events. The definition of hypertension in children and adolescents has been a statistical definition that is based on a body of normative data in children and adolescents. The upper 5 % of the normal BP distribution continues to be the basis on which hypertension in children and adolescents is defined (Falkner, 2011). Therefore, the definition of hypertension in childhood is systolic and/or diastolic BP that is $>95^{th}$ percentile according to sex, age, and height (Redwine, 2012; Falkner, 2012).

This chapter will explore the importance of investigating the childhood and adolescence hypertension that may emerge in adult life and debate a prevalence, incidence and occurrence of hypertension in children and adolescents, addition to addressing the methods and instruments used to determine hypertension, risk factors, health promotion, education and treatment for hypertensive children and adolescents.

2. Prevalence, Incidence and Occurrence of Hypertension in Children and Adolescents

Hypertension is known to be a major cause of morbidity and mortality in the United States and in many other countries, and the long-term health risks to children with hypertension may be substantial, nowadays, pediatric hypertension is commonly observed. Because of that, many countries are development normative and consensus about the normal levels of BP in every phase of life.

The prevalence of pediatric hypertension worldwide is not known, due to regional differences in the definition of high BP, the distribution of reference BP data, and the BP measurement methodology (Falkner, 2010).

Due to the difficulty in establishing a consensus on BP values for children and adolescents was realized in 2004 the National High BP Education Program Working Group on High BP in Children and Adolescents (Fourth Report), in parallel with recent updated recommendations for the evaluation of elevated BP in adults (Chobanian et al., 2003), created a new designation of "prehypertension" to identify children at greatest risk for developing future hypertension. The definition for prehypertension replaced the term "high normal BP". The criteria defining prehypertension were also statistically based and reflected expert opinion. The BP category of prehypertension in both adults and children was designed to identify a group of individuals for whom targeted preventive efforts could be most beneficial.

Although primary hypertension is more commonly identified in adolescence than earlier in childhood, there is little information about the incident rates of hypertension in childhood. Within the National Childhood BP database, a segment of adolescents underwent BP measurement at intervals of 2 years and 4 years. An analysis of these data found that, among adolescents with prehypertension, 14% had developed hypertension 2 years later, which yielded an approximate incidence rate of 7% per year. A limitation of these data is that they were based on only a single BP measurement for BP classification. However, without repeated BP measurement sessions for participants classified as having hypertension in a single BP measurement session, it is not possible to make a clinical diagnosis of hypertension (Falkner et al., 2008).

In neonates, hypertension can be detected in 1 to 2.5 percent (both term and preterm infants) admitted to neonatal intensive care units. The clinician needs to be knowledgeable about normative BP values, the optimal method to measure BP in newborns, the underlying etiologies, and clinical manifestations, in order to identify and treat neonatal hypertension. In babies, the hypertension is usually caused by prematurity or problems with the kidneys or heart (Sun et al., 2007).

The worldwide prevalence of hypertension in children is highly variable (2-13%), depending on the methodology employed. In Brazil, for example, it is estimated that the prevalence of hypertension in children and adolescents is 4% and it is considered imperative the need for BP measurement from 3 years of age (Ministério da Saúde, 2006).

On the world stage, has been discussed the importance and necessity of the assessment, detection and tracking of elevated BP in children and pre-teens. Researches, worldwide, demonstrate the need for implementations and normative consensus about the normal levels of BP in every phase of life, and its relation to gender. Therefore, a study published by Fourth Report (2004), a work of the United States government, demonstrate that children's growth and development, 'crude' BP values (in mmHg) are not used for the diagnosis of hypertension of children aged 1–17 years. Instead, a more precise BP classification should be made using the tables with 90th, 95th, and 99th percentiles by child's gender, age, and height.

Based on the use of $\geq 95^{th}$ percentile to define hypertension, it would be expected that the prevalence of hypertension would be approximately 5%. However, due to the effects of accommodation and regression to the mean with repeated measures, the prevalence of hypertension is lower than 5% and had been expected to be from 1–3% following the recommended three separate measurements in children with an initial BP measurement $\geq 95^{th}$ percentile and the prevalence of prehypertension in childhood was not known (Falkner, 2010). Muntner et al. (2004) reported on an analysis of data from the National Health and Nutrition Examination Surveys (NHANES) that demonstrated childhood BP levels were increasing. The authors found that the increase in childhood BP levels were largely, but not entirely, due to the childhood obesity epidemic. Subsequently, another analysis of childhood data in NHANES and earlier surveys by Din-Dzietham et al. (2007), confirmed that in recent decades there has been an increase in prevalence of hypertension in children. According to current reports the prevalence of childhood hypertension ranges from 3 - 5 % in United States children with higher rates among minority adolescents.

Childhood hypertension is increasing, largely driven by the increasing prevalence of overweight and obesity, furthermore other factors are related with the development of hypertension in children and adolescents like family history of hypertension and an unhealthy lifestyle — a bad diet, stress, and insufficient physical activity. (Rodrigues, Abreu and Gouvêa, 2012). There are still others conditions strongly associated with arterial hypertension in adolescence as smoking, use of contraceptives, cocaine, amphetamines, alcohol, anabolic steroids, phenylpropanolamine and pseudoephedrine (nasal decongestant).

3. Methods and Instruments Used to Determine Hypertension in Children and Adolescents

The percentile values for BP obtained by auscultation in gender, age and height specific format for a large number of children and is widely accepted as the reference standard for normative BP values. (Kuczmarski et al., 2000). It has been accepted that hypertension is confirmed when SBP and / or DBP are greater than or equal to 95th percentile for sex, age and height percentile plus 5 mmHg in three separate occasions.

It is noteworthy also that the band called prehypertension should be identified and valued for the purpose of adopting preventive measures stringent. BP values $\geq 90^{th}$ percentile and $<95^{th}$ percentile characterize pre-hypertension; values that are included in this range and exceeding the limits of 120/80 mmHg should also be considered as pre-hypertension, complying with the same guidelines for adults. Figures 1 (for girls) and 2 (for boys) summarize the classification recommended BP in children and adolescents.

Age (years)	Blood Pressure Percentile	SBP (mmHg) Height Percentile				DBP (mmHg) Height Percentile			
		5th	25th	75th	95th	5th	25th	75th	95th
	90th	97	98	101	103	52	53	55	56
1	95th	100	102	105	107	56	57	59	60
	99th	108	109	112	114	64	65	66	67
	90th	100	102	104	106	61	62	64	65
3	95th	104	105	108	110	65	66	68	69
	99th	111	113	115	117	73	74	75	76
	90th	104	106	109	111	68	69	70	72
6	95th	108	110	113	115	72	73	74	76
	99th	115	117	120	122	80	80	82	83
	90th	110	112	114	116	72	72	74	75
9	95th	114	115	118	120	76	76	78	79
	99th	121	123	125	127	83	84	85	87
	90th	115	118	121	123	74	75	77	79
12	95th	119	122	125	127	78	80	82	83
	99th	126	129	133	135	86	88	90	91
	90th	127	130	134	136	80	81	83	84
17	95th	131	134	138	140	84	86	87	89
	99th	139	141	145	147	92	93	95	97

*The height percentiles were determined with standard growth curves.

Figure 1. BP levels for girls 1 to 17 years of age, according to height percentile (Fourth report, 2004).

Age (years)	Blood Pressure Percentile	SBP (mmHg) Height Percentile				DBP (mmHg) Height Percentile			
		5th	25th	75th	95th	5th	25th	75th	95th
	90th	94	97	100	103	49	51	53	54
1	95th	98	101	104	106	54	55	57	58
	99th	105	108	112	114	61	63	65	66
	90th	100	103	107	109	59	60	62	63
3	95th	104	107	110	113	63	64	66	67
	99th	111	114	118	120	71	72	74	75
	90th	105	108	111	113	68	69	71	72
6	95th	109	112	115	117	72	73	75	76
	99th	116	119	123	125	80	81	83	84
	90th	109	112	115	118	72	74	76	77
9	95th	113	116	119	121	76	78	80	81
	99th	120	123	127	129	84	86	88	89
	90th	115	118	121	123	74	75	77	79
12	95th	119	122	125	127	78	80	82	83
	99th	126	129	133	135	86	88	90	91
	90th	127	130	134	136	80	81	83	84
17	95th	131	134	138	140	84	86	87	89
	99th	139	141	145	147	92	93	95	97

*The height percentiles were determined with standard growth curves.

Figure 2. BP levels for boys 1 to 17 years of age, according to height percentile (Fourth report, 2004).

Thus, Body size is the most important determinant of BP in children and adolescents and the classification of BP is more accurate when the values are adjusted for height as well as age and gender to avoid misclassifying children at the extremes of normal growth (Fourth report, 2004; Rosner et al., 1993).

In many countries the BP percentile level that is used to define high BP in children varies somewhat from the United States definitions described above. High BP in the United

Kingdon is defined as BP above the 98th percentile for age (Jackson, Thalange and Cole, 2007). BP reference values have also been reported in Northern Europe and Asia (Munkhaugen et al., 2008; Sung et al., 2008). These reports describe a slightly higher BP level at the 95th percentile. However, all epidemiological reports on normative childhood BP data demonstrate a consistent and significant relationship of BP with age, height, and body weight throughout childhood (Fourth report, 2004).

The standard device for BP measurements both in clinical settings and epidemiological studies has been the Mercury manometer (sphygmomanometer). When a systematic measurement method is applied, the results obtained with the sphygmomanometer are comparable with electronic measurement devices. The procedure of BP measurement by auscultation requires a child to be seated with his back supported, feet on the floor, right arm supported, and cubital fossa at heart level (Netea et al., 2003). When using a sphygmomanometer, a stethoscope is placed over the brachial artery pulse, proximal and medial to the cubital fossa, below the bottom edge of the cuff (2 cm above the cubital fossa).

Regardless of the procedure, the right arm is preferred for measurement because of the possibility of coarctation of the aorta, which might lead to false (low) readings in the left arm. The selection of appropriate cuff size is very important.

By convention, an inflatable bladder width must be at least 40% of the child's arm circumference, and its length should cover 80% to 100% of the armcircumference (measured in themiddle between the olecranon and the acromion). If the bladder is too short the BP could be overestimated, since the pressure is not fully transmitted to the artery (Petrie, Samimy and Addy, 1986). Pediatricians warn that most practitioners use inadequate cuffs in children and adolescents and recommend child/pediatric cuffs to be used in children and adolescents according to the arm circumference (cm) (Amaral, R., Espinosa, C., Santos, T., Weselowski, T., Passos, S. D., 2007) (Figure 3).

4. Risk Factors for the Development of Hypertension in Children and Adolescents

Hypertension has been linked to cardiovascular diseases, stroke and kidney disease (Chobanian et al., 2003). The relationship between hypertension and risk of cardiovascular disease (CVD) is linear, progressive and continuous, in that the higher the BP, the greater the risk of CVD (Mancia et al., 2009). The medical management or control of BP is thought to reduce the risk of serious cardiovascular disease.

In obese or overweight adolescents, and the known early development of atherosclerosis in children, identification and treatment of BP in children is essential (Luma and Spiotta, 2006).

Cardiovascular diseases are a major cause of morbidity and premature mortality in men and women in the industrialized world and many developing countries (Hayman et al., 2004). The WHO (2009) indicates the leading global risks for mortality in the world are high BP (13% of global deaths), tobacco use (9%), high blood glucose (6%), physical inactivity (6%) and overweight or obesity.

Title Cuff	Arm circumference (cm)	Width of bag (cm)	Lenght of bag (cm)
Newborn	5 - 7.5	3	5
Infant	7.5 - 13	5	8
Children	13 - 20	8	13
Young Adult	17 - 24	11	17

Figure 3. Recommended dimensions of the bag inflatable cuff ("American Heart Association").

Yoshinaga et al. (2010) stated that little is known about the impact of having one CV risk factor on the other levels of other CV factors in the general adolescent population. The researchers hypothesized that when adolescents have one risk factor, the level of the other CV risk factors worsens simultaneously. A sample of 1,257 healthy adolescents (549 males and 708 females) aged 15-18 years were assessed using: risk factors of abdominal obesity, hypertension, raised triglyceride levels, decreased HDL cholesterol levels and hyperglycemia.

Overweight/obesity is an important hypertension risk factor in children, adolescents and adults and it is well-known childhood obesity can predict the cardiovascular risk in adulthood (Sun et al., 2008). It is estimated that 30% of children and adolescents with overweight/obesity have hypertension (Sorof et al., 2002). With increasing childhood obesity, there is increasingly early onset of atherosclerosis (McGill et al., 2000).In a study involving Hong Kong Chinese overweight children aged 9-12 years (mean Body mass index (BMI) 25 ± 3 kg/m^2); BMI was independently associated with impaired arterial endothelial function and increased carotid intimal medial thickness, which are early markers of atherosclerosis (Woo et al. 2004b). An important result from this study is that these obesity-related early vascular dysfunctions are partially reversible by lifestyle modifications (Woo et al. 2004a). Prevalence of childhood and adolescence overweight/obesity has marked variation among developed and developing countries. The prevalence of childhood and adolescence obesity has tripled between 1980 and 2000 in United States and doubled between 1985 and 1995 in Australia (Ogden et al., 2002).

Homeostatic assessment of insulin resistance (HOMA-IR) was used as a surrogate marker of insulin resistance. The levels of all CV risk factors and HOMA-IR significantly and simultaneously worsened when adolescents had one risk factor, in both genders. Having one risk factor indicated the development of other risk factors in adolescents, especially the development of abdominal obesity in male subjects was found to have a harmful effect on other CV risk factors.

They concluded that it is important to determine the presence or absence of CV risk factors before and/or during adolescence, because having one CV risk factor can indicate the start of an accumulation of CV risk factors in the general adolescent population.

Heart attacks and coronary heart disease (CHD) are primarily caused by atherosclerosis, where a narrowing and hardening of the arteries result from an accumulation of fat and cholesterol deposits called plaque. This narrowing, or blockage of the arteries stops the supply of blood to the heart and can cause a heart attack, heart failure or even cardiac arrest.

Atherosclerotic cardiovascular disease is described as a multi-factorial condition reflecting a lifelong pathological process that begins in childhood (Stary, 1989). Chronic disease and illness are commonly caused by exposure to risk factors many years prior to the onset of the condition. Dietary/ nutritional intake, consumption of alcohol and other substances, smoking, and inactivity are all behaviour patterns established during adolescence and have been linked to obesity and a number of illnesses that develop later in life (Kilty and Prentice, 2012).

Similarly to adults, family history of hypertension is associated with higher BP in children. Children who have parents or siblings who have heart disease are more likely to develop it themselves. They have a significantly greater likelihood of having a heart attack or stroke. Familial hypercholesterolemia and its accompanying biological defects are well characterized as a known risk for hypertension development.

Children's nutrition may play an important role in the regulation of BP. According to the US Fourth Report (2004), despite the lack of firm evidence about dietary intervention in children, it is generally accepted that hypertensive individuals can benefit from a dietary increase in fresh vegetables, fresh fruits, fiber, and nonfat dairy as well as a reduction of sodium. However, it has been demonstrated that children consuming fruits and vegetables and dairy products showed slower increase of SBP in childhood and have lower BP in adolescence.

In addition, salt intake is correlated to BP in children, independently from age, gender and nutritional status (Figure 5).

Essential hypertension often is linked toother risk factors that make up metabolic syndrome (MS) and can lead to cardiovascular disease. These risk factors for metabolic syndrome include low plasma high-density lipoprotein, elevated plasma triglycerides, abdominal obesity, and insulin resistance/hyperinsulinemia (Figure 5). The prevalence of metabolic syndrome among adolescents is between 4.2 and 8.4 percent. (Goodman et al., 2004). Triglycerides are strongly associated with the risk of developing atherosclerotic disease because they can deposit on the vessel wall and then start the process of low-density lipoprotein accumulation.

	Boys			**Girls**		
Percentile	**5-9 y**	**10-14 y**	**15-19 y**	**5-9 y**	**10-14 y**	**15-19 y**
Total Cholesterol (mg/dL)						
75th	168	173	168	177	171	176
90th	183	191	183	189	191	198
95th	186	201	191	197	205	208
Triglycerides (mg/dL)						
75th	85	74	88	74	85	85
90th	70	94	125	103	104	112
95th	85	111	143	120	120	126
LDL (mg/dL)						
75th	103	109	109	115	110	110
90th	117	123	123	125	126	129
95th	129	133	130	140	136	137

Figure 4. Total Cholesterol, triglycerides and low density lipoproteins (LDL) levels for boys and girls 5 to 19 years of age, according to height percentile (Emmanouilides et al., 2000).

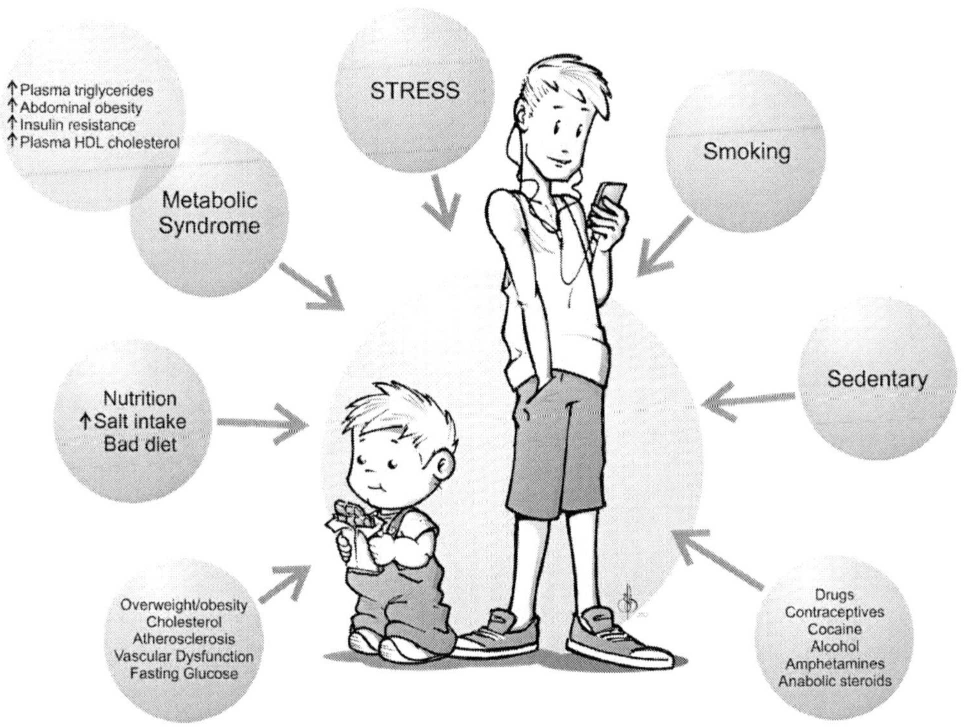

Figure 5. Hypertension risk factors in children and adolescents.

High levels of triglycerides are a key component of so-called MS (Johnson, et al., 1999; Santos et al., 2008; Cobayashi et al., 2010).

It is important to emphasize that when dyslipidemia begins in childhood, it tends to remain during growth, and that studies describe a direct relationship between total cholesterol levels in children and cardiovascular disease in adults (Forti et al., 1996). The variety of criteria for defining optimal lipid levels in adolescence makes it difficult to compare the results in the global literature. Therefore, the epidemiological goal for children should be, on average, 150 mg% for plasma cholesterol (Srinivasan, 1991).

In a review of studies conducted in 26 countries (1975 to 1996) involving 60,494 children and adolescents aged 2 to 19 years, Brotons et al. (1998) reported an average of 165 mg / dL for cholesterol, 60 mg / dL for HDL cholesterol and 67 mg / dL for triglycerides.

Although no well established in literature values the figure 4 shows total cholesterol, triglycerides and low density lipoproteins (LDL) levels for boys and girls 5 to 19 years of age, according to height percentile (Emmanouilides et al., 2000).

Physical activity is important for growth and development, weight and BP regulation. Increasing regular activity and decreasing sedentary activities such as watching television and playing video or electronic games have been found to be important components of pediatric obesity prevention and therefore, important to lowering of hypertension risk factors.

Identification of a child with multiple risk factors is important. The risk associated with any single identified factor is markedly affected by the intensity of coexistent risk factors.

As an approach to identifying multiple risk factors (Figure 5), a cardiovascular health profile can be completed for each child. Personal family history, smoking history (including passive smoking), BP percentiles, BMI percentile chart, serum cholesterol level, and level of fitness can be used to develop a composite estimate of coronary artery disease risk and to direct management. This profile graphically demonstrates to children and their families their risk factors for future coronary artery disease.

5. Health Promotion, Prevention, Risk Reduction and Education

Many hypertension risk factors are adopted by adolescents without awareness of their present and long term impacts on health or the potential development of heart disease. Adolescence is a life stage where the individual is still influenced by the family, but beginning to make independent choices in many areas to establish their own lifestyle habits, behaviors, values and beliefs. Most writers acknowledge that heart health education and screening can and should be initiated in childhood before adolescence begins. However, adolescence is a key point of entry, where risk factors can be made known not only to families, health practitioners, and educators, but to the individual adolescent directly so he or she can be potentially informed, empowered and motivated to make their own changes.

Conducting primary prevention of hypertension, beginning in early childhood and sustained through adolescence has been well supported by the extensive evidence from epidemiological, clinical, and laboratory studies conducted world-wide. Approaches to reduce and prevent cardiovascular disease can include *primary prevention* and health promotion for the general population before hypertension occurs; *secondary prevention* to identify those at risk and provide opportunities for change; and *tertiary prevention* to identify those with hypertension and associated risks such as diabetes and obesity and intervene (Kilty and Prentice, 2012).

Primary Prevention

Strategies to achieve, individuals, groups and populations should include information on heart health, holistic health and wellness. Therefore, awareness programs include risk monitoring data given to general, family physician adolescent, or community awareness and readiness to stimulate change.

Community settings for making contact with adolescents for health promotion and intervention have primarily been through the schools or health clinics and physicians' offices.

The school can be viewed as one of the most important settings in which social and psychological development occurs and it is likely that health and health behaviours may be associated with a relationship to school (Bond and Compas, 1989). Large numbers of adolescents can be reached for health education purposes through schools. The school is also an ideal venue for health promotion and education about cardiovascular risk.

Most schools have curriculum related well to health, health promotion and heart health. They also have teachers of science, health, sociology and physical education where content about cardiovascular health and risks are well suited.

Clinics and doctors' offices can also be viewed as potential places to health promotion for the general population before hypertension occurs. The only routine health intervention occurrences may be around immunization times that take place in teen years in some cultures.

Secondary Prevention

Should be carried out risk assessments, testing and screening methods that include testing and monitoring of BP, cholesterol, BMI calculations, waist circumference and physical activity. Also included should be specific lifestyle behavior change strategies that may include introducing specific interventions to reduce smoking, increase physical activity, improve nutrition, stop smoking; and reduce overweight and obesity. These approaches involve developing skills and behavioral changes.

It has been demonstrated that the mortality rate from cardiovascular disease is lower individuals who engage in regular exercise and there seems no doubt more regarding the improvement in quality of life achieved through a program of fitness. Childhood and adolescence appear to be periods for promoting physical activity habits of good behavior and prevention sedentary adulthood.

Therefore, prevention of cardiovascular disease is also a problem pediatric. Alerts have been issued on the needs of physical education programs in school, and community recreation facilities, since a greater fitness been related to lower cardiovascular risk profile in children and adolescents.

Obesity has deserved special attention to come usually accompanied by two notorious big risk factors: diabetes and hypertension. It is important, therefore, its control during childhood, since obesity acquired in this period of life, tend to persist into adulthood. Therefore, prevention of obesity in childhood is the best opportunity to introduce changes in lifestyle and thus further reducing cardiovascular morbidity and mortality.

Futhermore, cigarette smoking among adults primarily starts in adolescence and continues to be a major public health problem world-wide. Tobacco use is considered the number one individually preventable and modifiable cause of cancer and cardiovascular disease (Greenlund et al., 1996).

These lifestyle behavior change strategies highlight the necessity of placing adolescents in the forefront of preventive hypertension programs and should receive particular attention by healthcare authorities in order to minimize future hypertension attributed mortality rates.

Tertiary Prevention

Consultation, treatment and health counseling interventions for those who are identified with cardiovascular risks include retesting, monitoring, consultation, counseling or treatment provided in adolescent friendly environments.

These approaches require using effective referral, counseling, monitoring and treatment approaches that work best with adolescents. Some clinical recommendations are important for the detection and monitoring of children and adolescents with hypertension (Luma and Spiotta, 2006):

Clinical Recommendations

- BP should be checked routinely at every visit in children three years of age and older.
- Three separate readings of an elevated BP (greater than 90th percentile for age, height, and sex) on separate visits are needed to make the diagnosis of hypertension.
- Patients diagnosed with primary hypertension should have a comprehensive assessment for cardiovascular risk factors (lipid profile, fasting glucose, body mass index).
- Nonpharmacologic treatment (e.g., weight loss, dietary modifications, exercise) should be first-line therapy in patients with hypertension (95-99th percentile plus 5 mmHg).
- Pharmacologic treatment should be initiated in patients with hypertension (> 99th percentile plus 5 mmHg), symptomatic hypertension, when end-organ damage is present (left ventricular hypertrophy, retinopathy, proteinuria); and in hypertension (95-99th percentile plus 5 mmHg) when BP is unresponsive to lifestyle changes.

Treatment options for children and adolescents with hypertension (high BP) are similar to those available for adults. Because children typically have better general health, more physical reserve, and fewer formed habits than adults, considerable effort is spent on modifying lifestyle factors that can contribute to elevated BP (Williams et al., 2002).

The first step in treating children with hypertension is to determine whether the hypertension is primary (essential hypertension) or secondary (due to some underlying cause). This first step is vital because, in many cases, treating an underlying disorder can return the BP to normal without the need for additional treatment (Flynn and Daniels, 2006).

Essential hypertension rarely is found in children younger than 10 years and is a diagnosis of exclusion. Significant risk factors for essential hypertension include family history and increasing BMI. Some sleep disorders and black race can be potential risk factors for essential hypertension. Essential hypertension often is linked to other risk factors that make up metabolic syndrome and can lead to cardiovascular disease. These risk factors for metabolic syndrome include low plasma high-density lipoprotein, elevated plasma triglycerides, abdominal obesity, and insulin resistance or hyperinsulinemia (John et al., 2002).

Secondary hypertension is more common in children than in adults. It can present in adolescents, especially if they have physical findings not typically seen with essential hypertension. Renal disease is the most common cause of secondary hypertension in children (Buzzard and Lipshultz, 2001; Singh, Hurley, and Myers, 1992). Other causes include endocrine disease (e.g., pheochromocytoma, hyperthyroidism) and pharmaceuticals (e.g., oral contraceptives, sympathomimetics, some over-thecounter preparations, dietary supplements). Transient rise in BP, which can be mistaken for hypertension, is seen with caffeine use and certain psychological disorders (e.g., anxiety, stress). An underlying cause can be found in most children and adolescents with hypertension who are 1 to 18 years old. In the majority of cases the cause will be related to renal disease, although there are a number of others causes (Flynn, 2001; Bartosh and Aronson, 1999; Flynn, 2005) (Figure 6).

Nonpharmacologic and pharmacologic treatments are recommended based on the age of the child, the stage of hypertension, and response to treatment (Luma and Spiotta, 2006).

Age	Causes
1 - 6 years	Renal parenchymal disease; renal vascular disease; endocrine causes; coarctation of the aorta; essential hypertension.
6 - 12 years	Renal parenchymal disease; essential hypertension; renal vascular disease; endocrine causes; coarctation of the aorta; iatrogenic illness.
12 - 18 years	Essential hypertension; iatrogenic illness; renal parenchymal disease; renal vascular disease; endocrine causes; coarctation of the aorta.

Figure 6. Causes of childhood hypertension according to age group.

Nonpharmacologic treatment is recommended as initial therapy in children with essential hypertension. Attention should be given to weight, exercise, and diet, with the recognition that success increases with frequent reinforcement and encouragement.

Effective sodium restriction is not feasible in this age group. Obese adolescents have significant reductions in BP with weight loss, and the effect on BP is enhanced when exercise is incorporated into the weight-loss program. The degree of physical fitness has been shown to be inversely related to BP in grade-school children (Luma and Spiotta, 2006).

Reasons to initiate antihypertensive medication in children and adolescents include symptomatic hypertension, end-organ damage (e.g., LVH, retinopathy, proteinuria), secondary hypertension and hypertension that does not respond to lifestyle changes. In the absence of end-organ damage or co morbid conditions, the goal is to reduce BP to less than the 95th percentile for age, height, and sex. When end-organ damage or coexisting illness is present, a BP goal of less than the 90th percentile is recommended. Drug therapy is always an adjunct to no pharmacologic measures (Cutler, Follmann and Allender, 1997; Sorof et al., 2002; Wells et al., 2002).

Conclusion

Although the hypertension prevalence is far lower in children and adolescents than adults, increasing evidence indicates that essential hypertension begins to develop during the first two decades of life. Since even small increments in BP can have substantial effects on hypertension- related morbidity and mortality, greater attention to BP early in life may ultimately lead to considerable improvements in cardiovascular health.

In conclusion, hypertension is an increasing world health problem. In view of the substantial tracking of hypertension risk factors from adolescents to adulthood, there is an urgent need to intervene early with efficacious strategies to identify and treat hypertensive children and adolescents. The traditional hypertensive risk factors, namely overweight/obesity and family history, including lifestyle (a bad diet, stress, and insufficient physical activity) appear to be important, accounting for the dramatic recent changes in prevalence and would be of public health concern. Moreover, more intensive program for lifestyle modification and aggressive approach of pharmacological treatment should be considered in hypertensive children and adolescents.

Acknowledgments

The Fabricio Bragança da Silva the Postgraduate Program in Physiological Sciences, Federal University of Espírito Santo for creating the illustration made for this chapter.

References

Amaral, R., Espinosa, C., Santos, T., Weselowski, T., and Passos, S. D. (2007). Hipertensão arterial em pediatria: aspectos diagnósticos. *Perspectivas Médicas*, Vol. 18, No. 2, pp. 37-42.

Bartosh, S. M. and Aronson, A. J. (1999). Childhood hypertension. An update on etiology, diagnosis, and treatment. *Pediatr. Clin. North Am.*, Vol. 46, pp. 235-252.

Blumenthal, S., Epps, R. P., Heavenrich, R, Lauer, R. M., Lieberman, E., and Mirkin, B., (1977). Report of the task force on blood pressure control in children. *Pediatrics*, Vol. 59, pp. 797–820.

Bond, L. and Compas, B. (1989). *Primary prevention and promotion in the schools*. Newbury Park: Sage Pub.

Brotons, C., Ribera, A., Perich, R. M., Abrodos, D., Magana, P., Pablo, S., Terradas, D., Fernadez, F., and Permanyer, G. (1998). Worldwide distribution of blood lipidis and lipoproteins in childhood and adolescence: a review study. *Atherosclerosis*, Vol. 139, pp. 1-9.

Buzzard, C. J. and Lipshultz, S. E. (2001) High blood pressure in infants, children, and adolescents. In: *Primary pediatric care*. (4th edition). St. Louis, Mosby: Hoekelman, R. A., editor. pp. 1142–1149.

Chen, X. and Wang, Y. (2008). Tracking of blood pressure from childhood to adulthood: a systematic review and meta-regression analysis. *Circulation*, Vol. 117, No. 25, pp. 3171–80.

Chobanian, A. V., Bakris, G. L., Black, H. R., and et al. (2003). Seventh report of the joint national committee on prevention, detection, evaluation, and treatment of high blood pressure. *Hypertension*, Vol. 42, No.6, pp. 1206–52.

Cobayashi, F., Oliveira, F. L. C., Escrivão, M. A. M. S., Silveira, D., and Taddei, J. A. A. C. (2010). Obesity and Cardiovascular Risk Factors in Adolescents Attending Public Schools. *Arquivos Brasileiros de Cardiologia,* Vol. 95, No.2, pp. 200-206.

Cutler, J. A., Follmann, D. and Allender, P. S. (1997). Randomized trials of sodium reduction: an overview. *American Journal of Clinical Nutrition*, Vol. 65, pp. 643.

Din-Dzietham, R., Liu, Y., Bielo, M. V., and Shamsa, F. (2007). High blood pressure trends in children and adolescents in national surveys, 1963 to 2002. *Circulation*, Vol. 116, No.13, pp. 1488–1496.

Emmanouilides, G. C., Allen, H. D., Riemenschneider, T. A., and Gutgesell, H. P. (2000). Doenças do Coração na Criança e no Adolescente: Aterosclerose, Hipertensão e Doença Coronariana. Rio de Janeiro, RJ. Editora: Medsi Editora Médica e Científica Ltda.

Falkner, B. (2010). Hypertension in children and adolescents: epidemiology and natural history. *Pediatr. Nephrol.*, Vol. 25, No. 7, pp. 1219–1224.

Falkner, B. (2011). *Development of Blood Pressure Norms in Children: Pediatric Hypertension*, (Second edition). New York: Humana Press.

Falkner, B. (2012). Recent advances in pediatric hypertension. *Journal of clinical hypertension,* Vol. 14, No. 6, pp.345.

Falkner, B., Gidding, S. S., Portman, R., and Rosner, B. (2008). Blood pressure variability and classification of prehypertension and hypertension in adolescence. *Pediatrics*, Vol. 122, pp. 238–242.

Flynn, J. T. (2001). Evaluation and management of hypertension in childhood. *Prog. Pediatr. Cardiol.,* Vol. 12, pp. 177-188.

Flynn, J. T. (2005). Hypertension in adolescents. *Adolesc. Med. Clin.*, Vol. 16, pp. 11-29.

Flynn, J. T. and Daniels, S. R. (2006). Pharmacologic treatment of hypertension in children and adolescents. *Journal of Pediatrics*, pp. 149:746.

Forti, N., Diogo Giannini, S., Diament, J., Issa, J., Fukushima, J., Dal Bó, C. and Pereira Barretto, A. C. (1996). Fatores de risco para aterosclerose em filhos de pacientes com doença coronariana precoce. *Arquivos Brasileiros de Cardiologia*, Vol. 66, No. 3, pp. 119-123.

Goodman, E., Daniels, S. R., Morrison, J. A., Huang, B., and Dolan, L. M. (2004). Contrasting prevalence of and demographic disparities in the World Health Organization and National Cholesterol Education Program Adult Treatment Panel III definitions of metabolic syndrome among adolescents. *J. Pediatr.*, Vol.145, pp. 445-451.

Greenlund, K. J., Johnson, C., Wattigney, W., Bao, W., Webber, L. S., and Berenson, G. S. (1996). Trends in cigarette smoking among children in a southern community 1976-1994: The Bogalusa Heart Study. *American Journal of Pediatric Obesity,* Vol. 89, No. 8, pp. 1345-1348.

Hayman, L. L., Williams, C. L., Daniels, S. R., Steinberger, J., Paridon, S., Dennison, B. A., and McCrindle, B. W. (2004). Cardiovascular health promotion in the schools: a statement for health and education professionals and child health advocates from the Committee on Atherosclerosis, Hypertension, and Obesity in Youth (AHOY) of the Council on Cardiovascular Disease in the Young, American Heart Association. *Circulation*, Vol. 110, No. 15, pp.2266-2275.

Jackson, L. V., Thalange, N. K., and Cole, T. J. (2007). Blood pressure percentiles for Great Britain. *Arch. Dis. Child.*, Vol. 92, pp. 298–303.

John, M., Flack, M. D., Rosalind Peters, R. N., Vishal, C., Mehra, M. D., Samar, A., and Nasser, P. A. C. (2002). Hypertension in special populations. *Cardiol. Clin.*, Vol. 20, pp. 303–319.

Johnson, W. D., Kroon, J. J. M., Greenway, F. L., Bouchard, C., Ryan, D., and Katzmarzyk, P. T. (2009). Prevalence of risk factors for metabolic syndrome in adolescents national health and nutrition examination survey (NHANES), 2001-2006. *Archives of Pediatrics and Adolescent Medicine*, Vol. 163, No.4, pp. 371-377.

Kelishadi, R., Zadegan, N. S., Naderi, G. A., Asgary, S. and Bashardoust, N. (2002). Atherosclerosis risk factors in children and adolescents with or without family history of premature coronary artery disease. *Medical Science Monitor,* Vol. 8, No.6, pp. 425-429.

Kilty, H. L. and Prentice, D. (2012). Cardiovascular risk factors: Early Identification of Cardiovascular Risk Factors in Adolescents and Follow-Up Intervention Strategies. Rijeka, Croatia: Silvia Vlase.

Kuczmarski, R. J., Ogden, C. L., Grummer-Strawn, L. M., and et al. (2000) CDC growth charts: United States. *Adv. Data*, Vol. 314, pp.1–27.

Lloyd-Jones, D., Adams, R., Carnethon, M.,Wasserthiel-Smoller, Wong, N., Wylie-Rosett, J. and Hong, Y., Rosamond, Sacco, R., Sorlie, P., Stafford, R., Steinberger, J., Thom, T., Meigs, S., Mozaffarian, D., Nichol, G., O'Donnell, C., Roger, G., Wayne, Kittner, S., Lackland, D., Lisabeth, L., Marelli, A., McDermott, M., Greenlund, J. K., Haase, N., Hailpern, S., Ho, M., Howard, V., and Kissela, B. (2009). Heart Disease and Stroke Statistics--2009 Update: A Report From the American Heart (WHO). *Circulation*, Vol. 119, pp. 480-486.

Luma, G. B. and Spiotta, R. T. (2006). Hypertension in Children and Adolescents. *Am. Fam. Physician*, Vol. 73, No. 9, pp. 1558-1568.

Mancia, G., Laurent, S., Agabiti-Rosei, E., Ambrosioni, E., Burnier, M., Caulfield, M. J., Cifkova, R., Clément, D., Coca, A., Dominiczak, A., Erdine, S., Fagard, R., Farsang, C., Grassi, G., Haller, H., Heagerty, A., Kjeldsen, S. E., Kiowski, W., Mallion, J. M., Manolis, A., Narkiewicz, K., Nilsson, P., Olsen, M. H., Rahn, K. H., Redon, J., Rodicio, J., Ruilope L., Schmieder, R. E., Struijker-Boudier, H. A., van Zwieten, P. A., Viigimaa, M., and Zanchetti, A. (2009). Reappraisal of European guidelines on hypertension management: a European Society of Hypertension Task Force document. *J. Hypertens*. Vol. 27, No. 11, pp. 2121-2158.

McGill, H. C. Jr., McMahan, C. A., Herderick, E. E., Malcom, G. T., Tracy, R. E., and Strong, J. P. (2000). Origin of atherosclerosis in childhood and adolescence. *Am. J. Clin. Nutr*. Vol. 72, No. 5, pp. 1307S-1315S.

Ministério da Saúde (2006). Hipertensão arterial sistêmica, saúde da família. Cadernos de Atenção Básica, No.15, Brasília, Distrito Federal.

Munkhaugen, J., Lydersen, S., Wideroe, T-E., and Hallan, S. (2008). Blood pressure reference values in adolescents: methodological aspects and suggestions for Northern Europe tables based on the Nord-Trondelag Health Study II. *J. Hypertens*., Vol. 26, pp. 1912–1918.

Munter, P. H. J., Cutler, J. A., Wildman, R. P., and Welton, P. K. (2004). Trends in blood pressure among children and adolescents. *JAMA*, Vol. 291, pp. 2107–2113.

National High Blood Pressure Education Program Working Group on High Blood Pressure in Children and Adolescents (2004). The fourth report on the diagnosis, evaluation, and treatment of high blood pressure in children and adolescents. *Pediatrics*, Vol. 114, pp. 555– 576.

Netea, R. T., Lenders, J. W., Smits, P., and Thien, T. (2003). Both body and arm position significantly influence blood pressure measurement. *J. Hum. Hypertens., Vol*. 17, No. 7, pp. 459-62.

Ogden, C. L., Flegal, K. M., Carroll, M. D., and Johnson, C. L. (2002). Prevalence and trends in overweight among US children and adolescents, 1999-2000. *JAMA*, Vol. 288, No. 14, pp.1728-1732.

Petrie, H. L., Samimy, M. and Addy, A. L. (1986). Compressible separated flows. *AIAA J.*, Vol. 24, No. 12, pp.1971–1978.

Redwine, K. M. and Falkner, B (2012). Progression of Prehypertension to Hypertension in Adolescents. *Curr. Hypertens. Rep.*, Vol. 14, pp. 619–625.

Redwine, K. M., Acosta, A. A., Poffenbarger, T., Portman, R. J., and Samuels, J. (2012). Development of hypertension in adolescents with pre-hypertension. *J. Pediatr.*, Vol. 160, No1, pp. 98–103.

Rodrigues, A. N., Abreu, G. R. and Gouvêa, S. A. (2012). Cardiovascular risk factors: Cardiovascular Risk Investigation: When Should It Start?. Rijeka, Croatia: Silvia Vlase.

Rosner, B., Prineas, R. J., Loggie, J. M., and Daniels, S. R. J. (1993). Blood pressure nomograms for children and adolescents, by height, sex, and age, in the United States. *Pediatrics*, Vol. 123, No. 6, pp. 871.

Santos, M. G., Pegoraro, M., Sandrini, F., and Macuco, E. C. (2008). Fatores de Risco no Desenvolvimento da Aterosclerose na Infância e Adolescência. *Arquivos Brasileiros de Cardiologia*, Vol. 90, No.4, pp. 301-308.

Singh, H. P., Hurley, M. and Myers, T. G. (1992). Neonatal hypertension: incidence and risk factors. *Am. J. Hypertens.*, Vol. 5, pp. 51–55.

Sorof, J. M., Cargo, P., Graepel, J., and et al. (2002). Beta-blocker/thiazide combination for treatment of hypertensive children: a randomized double-blind, placebo-controlled trial. *Pediatric Nephrology*, Vol. 17, pp. 345.

Sorof, J. and Daniels, S. (2002). Obesity hypertension: a problem of epidemic proportions. *Hypertension*, Vol. 40, pp. 441 447.

Srinivasan, S. R. (1991). Racial (black-white) differences in serum lipoprotein (a)–distribution ant its relation to parental myocardial infarction in children: the Bogalusa Heart Study. *Circulation*, Vol. 84, pp. 160-167.

Stary, H. C. (1989). Evolution and progression of atherosclerotic lesions in coronary arteries of children and young adults. *Arteriosclerosis*. Vol. 9, pp. I19–I32.

Sun, S. S., Grave, G. D., Siervogel, R. M., Pickoff, A. A., Arslanian, S. S., and Daniels, S. R. (2007). Systolic blood pressure in childhood predicts hypertension and metabolic syndrome later in life. *Pediatrics*, Vol. 119, No.2, pp. 237.

Sun, S. S., Liang, R., Huang, T. T., Daniels, S. R., Arslanian, S., Liu, K., Grave, G. D., and Siervogel, R. M. (2008). Childhood obesity predicts adult metabolic syndrome: the Fels Longitudinal Study. *J. Pediatr.*, Vol. 152, pp. 191-200.

Sung, R. Y. T., Choi, K. C., So H-K., Nelson, E. A. S., Li, A. M., Kwok, C. W. L, Tong, G. N., Mak, K. H., Ng, P. C., and Fok, T. F. (2008). Oscillometrically measured blood pressure in Hong Kong Chinese children and associations with anthropometric parameters. *J. Hypertens.*, Vol. 26, pp. 678–684.

Wells, T., Frame, V., Soffer, B., and et al. (2002). A double-blind, placebo-controlled, dose-response study of the effectiveness and safety of enalapril for children with hypertension. *Journal of Clinical Pharmacology*, Vol. 42, pp. 870.

Williams, C. L., Hayman, L. L., Daniels, S. R., and et al. (2002). Cardiovascular health in childhood: A statement for health professionals from the Committee on Atherosclerosis, Hypertension, and Obesity in the Young (AHOY) of the Council on Cardiovascular Disease in the Young. American Heart Association. *Circulation*, pp. 106:143.

Woo, K. S., Chook, P., Yu, C. W., Sung, R. Y., Qiao, M., Leung, S. S., and et al. (2004). Effects of diet and exercise on obesity-related vascular dysfunction in children. *Circulation*, Vol. 109, pp. 1981-1986.

Woo, K. S., Chook, P., Yu, C. W., Sung, R. Y., Qiao, M., Leung. S. S., and et al. (2004). Overweight in children is associated with arterial endothelial dysfunction and intima-media thickening. *Int. J. Obes. Relat. Metab. Disord.*, Vol. 28, pp. 852-857.

Yoshinaga, M., Ichiki, T., Tanaka, Y., Hazeki, D., and et al. (2010). Prevalence of childhood obesity from 1978 to 2007 in Japan. *Pediatrics International*, Vol. 52, No. 2, pp. 213-217.

In: Arterial Hypertension
Editors: Marten Vosler and Siemen Weber

ISBN: 978-1-62417-852-8
© 2013 Nova Science Publishers, Inc.

Chapter 6

Target Organ Damage in Hypertensive Patients

Paolo Calabrò**, Francesco Natale, Giuseppe Limongelli, Claudia Concilio, Chiara Cirillo, Chiara Granato, Alessandro Siciliano, Alessandro Ranieri, Baniamino Casillo, Pina Elvira Russo, Lucia Riegler, Michele Adolfo Tedesco, Maria Giovanna Russo and Raffaele Calabrò

Division of Cardiology, Second University of Naples,
A.O. dei Colli Monaldi Hospital, Naples, Italy

Abstract

Hypertension should be considered a major risk factor for an array of cardiovascular and related diseases. Both systolic and diastolic blood pressures show a graded independent relationship with heart failure, peripheral artery disease and end stage renal disease. The 2003 ESH-ESC Guidelines emphasized that diagnosis and management of hypertension should be related to quantification of total (or global) cardiovascular risk. This concept is based on the fact that only a small fraction of the hypertensive population has an elevation of blood pressure alone, with the great majority exhibiting additional cardiovascular risk factors. Due to the importance of subclinical organ damage as an intermediate stage in the continuum of vascular disease and as a determinant of total cardiovascular risk, signs of organ involvement should be sought carefully by appropriate techniques:

- heart: electrocardiography and echocardiography should be part of all routine assessment of subjects with high BP;
- blood vessels: ultrasound scanning of carotid arteries is recommended when detection of vascular hypertrophy or asymptomatic atherosclerosis is deemed useful;

* Corresponding Author: Dr. Paolo Calabrò, MD, FESC; Division of Cardiology, Second University of Naples, A.O. dei Colli Monaldi Hospital, Naples, Italy; paolo.calabro@unina2.it

- kidney: diagnosis of hypertension-related renal damage is based on a reduced renal function or an elevated urinary excretion of albumin;
- fundoscopy: examination of eye grounds is only recommended in severe hypertensives;
- brain: silent brain infarcts, lacunar infarctions, microbleeds and white matter lesions are not infrequent in hypertensives, and can be detected by MRI or CT.

It is now clear that the stratification of cardiovascular risk through the assessment of organ damage is important for treating and reducing the risk of cardiovascular disease.

Vascular Tissue

Endothelial Dysfunction

The endothelium is an early target of cardiovascular risk factors and cardiovascular diseases like arterial hypertension. endothelium has a key role because of its capacity to respond to numerous autocrine and paracrine stimuli and to mechanical factors like shear stress, but also from the pathophysiological consequences of endothelial dysfunction on vasomotor tone, arterial stiffness, arterial remodeling, and inflammation, all of which are factors that play a critical role in atherosclerosis and target-organ damage [1].

Endothelial dysfunction is the earliest measurable alteration in arterial wall function that can be measured *in vivo*. Early detection of endothelial dysfunction in EH is possible by measuring hemodynamic changes by ultrasound, by occlusive plethysmography, and measuring circulating markers of defective EC function (ET-1, adhesion molecules, tumor necrosis factor, von Willebrand's factor, plasminogen activator inhibitor-1, asymmetric dimethyl L-arginine) [2,3,4,5].

Endothelial dysfunction defines pathological modifications of coagulation, inflammatory, vascular growth regulation properties, deregulation of vascular remodeling which includes production of nitrogen oxide (NO) and other different vasoactive substances (endothelin-1, thromboxane A2, and angiotensin II) [7]. The concept of endothelium dysfunction in literature it is often described as an impairment of endothelium-dependent vasodilatation caused by decreased NO bioavailability in the vessel wall [8].

It has been demonstrated that hypertensive patients present endothelial dysfunction [9, 10,11]. In 1991 Moncada et al shown that under basal conditions the whole-body NO bioavailability is reduced in hypertensive patients.

These patients have shown to have impaired endothelium-dependent vasodilative response of the peripheral resistance arteries to molecules such as acetylcholine which is a NO stimulant, but not to nitroprusside, an endothelium-independent vasodilator [12].

Endothelium-dependent vasodilation is markedly impaired in the coronary microvessels of patients with hypertension and ventricular hypertrophy. Loss of this vasodilator mechanism may contribute to disordered coronary flow regulation and the ischemic manifestations of hypertensive heart disease [4]. Evidence on defective NO-mediated vasodilation in the etiopathogenesis of arterial hypertension has been further strengthened by data its recognition in still normotensive children of hypertensive parents [4].

The relationship between Endothelium dysfunction and hypertension has been studied widely and it is reasonable to hypnotize that they are causally related and it seems that endothelial dysfunction deteriorates further in evolving hypertension. The reduction of NO bioavailability has been related to increased circulating level of the endogenous NO synthase inhibitor [2].

An important role in development of endothelium injury in EH is played by Oxidative stress. Oxidative stress is defined as imbalance between production of reactive oxygen species (ROS) and antioxidants that neutralize them [13]. Increased formation of ROS determine reduced NO bioavailability. Increased production of ROS has been observed in human hypertension [14,15]. Increased production of vascular ROS, especially superoxide anion (O2–) contributes significantly to functional and morphological alterations in hypertension [16]. Superoxide production and low NO bioavailability lead to endothelial dysfunction and hypertrophy of vascular cells which promotes atherosclerosis. Experimental data indicate an enhanced superoxide generation as a result of the activation of vascular NAD(P)H oxydase in hypertension [17]. Renin-angiotensin-aldosterone system (RAAS) is the best known regulator of blood pressure and one of the most important causal factor of target organ damage. Apart from circulating RAAS, recent evidence shows that tissue RAAS also exists and is generated in the vessel wall, the heart and the kidney. Constituents of RAAS could enter the endothelium or could originate from it [18].

The role of angiotensin II in humoral modulation is very well known. Angiotensin II modifies the vascular tone either directly by activation angiotensin 1 (AT1) receptors in vessel wall myocytes or indirectly by stimulation of norepinephrine secretion from the nerve endings [19,20]. Whereas angiotensin's hemodynamic effects in acute are useful, its cronic elevation could have severe consequences: Angiotensin II can cause endothelial dysfunction, vascular stiffness and accelerated atherogenesis independently from BP [20]. in hypertension secretion of Angiotensin is increased due to pulsatile stretch of arterial wall leading to increased local effects of AT1 receptors. The RAAS system affects vessel integrity not only through Angiotensin II, but Aldosterone plays a role in endothelium dysfunction, fibrosis and inflammation of arterial wall due to systemic electrolytes and hemodynamic imbalance [21,22].

Furthermore overactivation of RAAS may determine ET-1 production and activation of angiotensin-converting enzyme (ACE), which splits bradykinin, an important endothelium-derived relaxing factor [23]. There are some measures to prevent endothelian dysfunction or even to improve endothelial function. Management of risk factors such as hypercholesterolemia, hypertension can improve endothelial function and prevent damages [24,25]. Studies have demonstrated that endothelial dysfunction can be improved by substances with protective effects on endothelium such as L arginine, antioxidants or by life habits changings (exercise, diet).

Morphological Changes of the Large Atherosclerotic Arteries

Essential hypertension is an important risk factor for atherosclerosis. Pathogenesis of atherosclerotic plaque is well known. Endothelium is considered an autocrine-paracrine organ with a central role in many physiological processes. These include the regulation of the vascular tone, platelet activity, hemocoagulation and cell proliferation, which are all part of the vascular homeostasis. Endothelial cells are capable of answering both to hemodynamic stimuli (shear stress, pressure variations) and specific mediators (hormones, peptides, local metabolites, platelet-derived factors) by producing different biologically active substances.

Endothelial-derived factors are classified in two groups:

- substances with a vasodilatative, antiproliferative, antiplatelet or antithrombotic action (nitric oxide, prostacyclins, endothelium-derived hyperpolarizing factor); which are prevalent in the normal endothelium;
- substances with a vasoconstrictive, pro-mitotic or prothrombotic action (endothelin-1, prostaglandin H2, thromboxane A2, angiotensin II, oxygen free radicals).

Nitric oxide is the most important of the endothelium-derived vasoactive factors. Other than being a vasodilatative substance, it also has antithrombotic activity and inhibits platelet aggregation, the production of endothelin, the migration and the proliferation of smooth muscle cells, the expression of adhesion molecules, and the adhesion of circulating monocytes.

Physiologically, there is a balance between the endothelium's vasodilatative/ antiproliferative and vasoconstrictive/pro-mitotic actions with a prevalence of the effects mediated by nitric oxide. In the endothelial dysfunction there is a reduction to release of NO and the prevalence of vasoconstrictive/pro-mitotic actions. It has been proposed that various interrelated molecular and cellular processes, including inflammation, may be a consequence of mechanical and chemical damage of the endothelium. This can be determined by different risk factors, such as hypertension [26,27,28,29].

A recent hypothesis is that target organ damage of essential hypertension is characterized in the first place by endothelial dysfunction [27, 28, 29, 30], which determines development and progression of the atherosclerotic plaque by releasing substances with a vasoconstrictive, pro-mitotic or prothrombotic action. Subsequently rupture of the fibrous cap of the plaque and thrombus formation is the event that leads to development of the majority of myocardial infarctions [31]

It's infrequent to find EH alone in an individual patient, more often atherosclerosis risk factors tend to cluster. Metabolic syndrome is characterized by: glucose intolerance, dyslipidemia, obesity, a pro-thrombotic and a pro-inflammatory state [32,33,34,35,36,37] Patients affected by metabolic syndrome present an increased risk of diseases related to atherosclerosis like coronary heart disease, peripheral vascular disease and stroke [38]. Ultrasounds are used to evaluate precocious alterations of the vasal wall and their development over time by studying the intima-media thickness (IMT) [39]. IMT is evaluated one cm under the common carotid artery's bifurcation. The cut-off is 0,75-1,00mm. Carotid arteries enable us to estimate the progression of arterial disease because of the tight associations between atherosclerotic changes in their wall and those in other parts of the circulation, especially coronary arteries [40]. Several studies have shown a significant relationship between carotid arterial IMT and cardiovascular risk factors [41,42]. Furthermore, healthy normotensive offspring of parents with EH may present thicker IMT, implying a possible hereditary transmission of the morphological alterations [43].

Interventional studies have shown the relation between IMT and EH. ELSA (European Lacidipine Study on Atherosclerosis), one of the most important of them, assessed IMT in EH patients. It demonstrated that the slowing of progression of the thickening could be achieved only by some drugs irrespective of the comparable lowering of the BP [44]. Recently, we got strong evidence that IMT is not only an independent risk factor for cardiovascular events, but also a better predictor of events than other known single conventional risk factors. Surrogate measurements of arterial stiffness, like pulse pressure and pulse wave velocity, indicate that it increases both with age and in certain disease states that are themselves associated with increased cardiovascular risk. These include hypertension, diabetes mellitus and hypercholesterolemia [45]. Arterial stiffness may be measured using different techniques, mainly ultrasound based.

The most commonly used parameter in detecting central arterial stiffness is applanation tonometry pulse wave velocity [46]. Arterial stiffening has been associated to the development of isolated systolic hypertension and heart diseases which determine increased cardiovascular morbidity and mortality [46].

Kidney

EH one of the main causes of chronic kidney disease, even though the mechanisms responsible are still partly unknown [47]. It has been hypothesized that EH determines hypertensive nephropathy. Initially, the self regulation systems of the pre- and postglomerular resistance vessels keep the blood pressure normal in the glomerular capillaries. In time, the vasoconstriction of the afferent arterioles may cause: endothelial dysfunction of the preglomerular arteries, myointimal hyperplasia and hyalinosis of the afferent, interlobular and interlobar blood vessels. The consequence is a vascular stenosis responsible of hyschaemia and global glomerulosclerosis. The different alterations have a different impact in determining evolution of the nephropaty depending on the severity of the hypertension [48,49]. An increase in RAAS activity may play a relevant role in the pathomorphological modifications found in hypertensive nephrosclerosis [50]. It as been shown that the evolution of chronic nephropathy may be delayed or interrupted using ACE inhibitors, AT1 receptor blockers (ARBs) and direct renin inhibitors such as aliskiren [51,52].

Elevated blood-pressure levels are associated with CKD progression. In treating patients with CKD it is of primary importance to maintain optimal salt and volume balance to achieve blood-pressure goals. Furthermore, drugs affecting renin-angiotensin-aldosterone axis are a valuable adjunct to therapy monitoring changes in serum creatinine and electrolyte levels after their administration.

Even slight reductions of renal function may be considered as independent risk factors for developing cardiovascular disease [53,54]. Uncontrolled hypertension is associated with increased risk of cardiovascular morbidity and mortality. The risk of cardiovascular mortality doubles for each 20 mmHg increase in systolic blood pressure and 10 mmHg increase in diastolic blood pressure above 'normal' blood pressure levels of 115/75 mmHg.[55] Uncontrolled blood pressure in CKD patients is associated with cardiovascular morbidity and mortality. [56]. There is a strong connection between blood pressure, cardiovascular disease risk and risk of CKD in a 15-year follow-up study of approximately 12,000 hypertensive individuals at multiple Veterans Affairs centers in the USA [57]. Poorly controlled blood pressure was a clear risk factor for the development of CKD and cardiovascular complications and lowering of blood pressure was associated with a reduced risk of developing CKD.

A decrease in systolic blood pressure of >2 mmHg after treatment was associated with a marked decrease in the relative risk of developing ESRD. Early signs of hypertensive nephropathy are reduced glomerular filtration rate and mild albuminuria, both of which can be easily evaluated. Albuminuria is a consequence of an increase in the glomerular permeability that is caused by functional and morphological alterations [58]. Increasing albuminuria correlates with an exponential increase in the risk of developing chronic renal failure and cardiovascular complications [59].

Antihypertensive therapy can prevent the progression of albuminuria and chronic renal failure improving renal and cardiovascular prognosis [60]. Treatment with ARB (losartan) is associated with less cardiovascular complications, as demonstrated in the LIFE study's reduction of albuminuria in hypertensive patients with left ventricular (LV) hypertrophy compared to atenonol [61]. Although recent results of ONTARGET study show that in people at high vascular risk, telmisartan's effects on major renal outcomes are similar to ramipril. Although combination therapy reduces proteinuria to a greater extent than monotherapy, overall it worsens major renal outcomes. [62].

Heart

Hypertensive Heart Disease

Manifestations of cardiac organ damage in patients with EH are:

- left ventricular hyperthrophy
- diastolic dysfunction
- reduced coronary flow reserve

All these pathological alterations are interrelated and may result in CAD, heart failure and arrhythmia [63].

Abnormaliers in Left Ventricular Diastolic Function

Diastolic dysfunction can be defined as a reduction of the heart's ventricular filling during the diastole with or without alterations of the systolic ejection fraction. It is thought to represent an important intermediate between hypertension and heart failure, particularly in heart failure with normal ejection fraction [63].

In hypertensive patients abnormalities in the left ventricular filling can be diagnosed before any alteration of the left ventricular ejection fraction are evident. The diastolic dysfunction is a negative prognostic factor for both the cardiovascular patologies and patient's survival rate. Several studies have shown a mortality rate from 13% to 23% (average follow up of 37 months).

Diastolic filling abnormalities in hypertensive heart disease result from a delayed LV relaxation. In later stages reduced LV compliance is observed as well due to increased myocardial fibrosis [64]. Factors influencing fibrosis may be systemic/local RAAS or parts of it and ET-1 [65,66]. The most commonly used noninvasive tool for assessment of cardiac function is now echocardiography.

Detailed information can be obtained by standard pulsed Doppler echocardiography and from recent developed tissue Doppler-, strain rate- and speckle tracking imaging [67]. The four chamber apical projection is used to assess diastolic function. The sample volume of the pulsed Doppler is placed at the apex of the open leaflet mitral valve. Then, in patients with a sinusal rythm, the early filling protodiastolic wave (E) and atrial contraction wave (A). The speed of E depends on the atrial pressure upon the opening of the mythralic valve, active ventricular relaxation and atrial compliance.

The "Deceleration E-Time" (DET) is the time required by the E wave to return to baseline values after its speed peak. It is influenced by the speed at which the endoventricular protodiastolic pressure increases and is correlated to the left ventricular compliance and active ventricular relaxation. The A wave mainly depends on ventricular compliance and the left atrium's contractile strength.

Alterations of the left ventricular compliance and relaxation are common in hypertensive patients.

Possible patterns are:

- normal pattern: E wave >A wave; DET =200ms;
- pseudonormal pattern: E/A between 1 and 2; DET >150ms;
- altered relaxation patter: E wave <A wave; DET >250ms;
- restrictive pattern: E/A <2; DET <150ms.

Left Ventricular Hypertrophy in Hypertensive Patients

In patients with sustained hypertension the heart develops concentric hypertrophy that is characterized by left ventricular walls thickening. Hypertrophic process is initially adaptive and enables the heart to neutralize wall stress associated with increased impedance to ventricular emptying (afterload), but then it is accompanied by a series of maladaptive changes that occur in the extracellular matrix as well as in cardiac myocytes. Despite its pathogenetic mechanisms has not been completely understood, LV hypertrophy is responsible of an increased incidence of myocardial infarction, heart failure, ventricular arrhythmias and sudden cardiac death [68].

Genetic background seems to play a role in evolving hypertension since hypertrophy can be found in prehypertensive period of evolving hypertension [69]. Other times hypertrophy develops more slowly and it depends from various components of cardiomyocytes response to pressure overload. One of them is a slowing of maximum shortening velocity (Vmax) because normally it allows the cardiac contraction at a normal energy cost. Beside, pressure overload causes multiplication of contractile unit and increased cell size preserving LV chamber function [70].

Another component of the cardiomyocyte response is a shift in substrate oxidation from fatty acids (FAs) toward carbohydrates [71]. These pathophysiological mechanisms seem to be due to re-expression of the cardio myocyte fetal gene program. [72]. An increasing number of genes have been described, including members of the RAAS system, the type A human natriuretic peptide receptor gene, protein G gene affecting the Na+/H+ exchanger, as well as genes related to contractility and function such as the myosin-binding protein C and genes involved in the β- adrenergic system [8]. Among them, the most strongly associated with LV hypertrophy is the polymorphism of genes that encode components of the RAAS system [73].

A frequent complication of established hypertension is reduced coronary vasodilation reserve. It may present itself in the absence of angiographic signs or demonstrable atherosclerotic disease [74] and it could be even detected in hypertensive patients that do not present LV hypertrophy [75]. There is evidence of a link between endothelial dysfunction and microvascular angina (syndrome X).

Microvascular angina in patients that present endothelial dysfunction in the resistance vessels is probably due to diminished formation of NO. Changes in morphology of small vessels and the discrepancy between increased LV mass and blood supply are another pathophysiological mechanism responsible of reduced coronary reserve in small arteries [76]. Increased media/lumen ratio, rarefaction of blood vessels in the myocardium) represent adaptations to an increased hemodynamic load imposed by increased BP [77].

Hypertrophy can be evaluated by different methods. In all hypertensive patients should be practiced an ECG, but it is more cost-effective and has high specificity and lower sensitivity. The gold standard is Echocardiography that can estimate a patient's left ventricular mass and assess for other morphological cardiac abnormalities. Many antihypertensive drugs are available and every class could diminish LV mass but with different efficacy. ACE inhibitors and ARBs seem to be superior to other classes of antihypertonic agents [78].

It has been demonstrated that reduction of the LV mass is associated with reduced cardiovascular risk [79] and that benefits from ACE inhibitors and ARBs therapy tended to be greater than those expected from a decrease in BP. These effects "beyond BP control" maybe responsible for the protective properties of these drugs [80,81,82].

Conclusion

Endothelial dysfunction has a key role in the pathogenesis of essential hyperthension. Abnormalities in endothelial function can lead to functional and morphological changes in small resistance vessels and are thought to be both cause and consequence of hypertensive disease. Target organ damage in resistence vessels, kidney and heart are the consequence of elevated blood pressure.

Target organ damage can be evaluated by non-invasive ultrasounds based methods. There isn't currently effective treatment for target organ damage. It is important to treat hypertension in the early stages, when preventive measures and antihypertensive therapy (preferably angiotensin-converting enzyme inhibitors and angiotensin receptor blockers) are most effective.

References

[1] C. Thuillez and V. Richard Targeting endothelial dysfunction in hypertensive subjects. *Journal of Human Hypertension* 2005. Jun;19 Suppl 1:S21-5.

[2] Achan V, Broadhead M, Malaki M, et al. Asymmetric dimethylarginine causes hypertension and cardiac dysfunction in humans. *Arterioscler Thromb Vasc Biol* 2003; 23: 1455–59.

[3] Devaraj S, Xu DY, Jialal I.C-reactive protein increases plasminogen activator inhibitor-1 expression and activity in human aortic endothelial cells: implications for the metabolic syndrome and atherothrombosis. *Circulation.* 2003 Jan 28;107(3):398-404.

[4] Treasure CB, Klein LJ, Vita JA, et al. Hypertension and left ventricular hypertrophy are associated with impaired endothelium-mediated relaxation in human coronary resistence vessels. *Circulation* 1993; 87: 86–93.

[5] Yang Z, Arnet U, Bauer E, et al. Thrombin-induced endothelium-dependent inhibition and direct activation of platelet-vessel wall interaction. Role of prostacyclin, nitric oxide, and thromboxane A2. *Circulation* 1994; 89: 2266–72.

[6] Žižek B, Poredoš P, Videčnik V (2001a). Endothelial dysfunction in hypertensive patients and in normotensive offspring of subjects with essential hypertension. *Heart*; 85: 215.

[7] Moncada S, Palmer RM, Higgs EA. Nitric oxide: Physiology, Pathophysiology, and Pharmacology. *Pharmacol Rev* 1991; 43: 109–42.

[8] Poredoš P. Endothelial dysfunction and cardiovascular disease. *Pathophysiol Haemost Thromb*; 32: 274–7.

[9] Egashira K, Suzuki S, Hirooka Y, et al. Impaired endothelium-dependent vasodilation of large epicardial and resistance coronary arteries in patients with essential hypertension. Different responses to acetylcholine and substance P. *Hypertension* 1995; 25: 201–6.

[10] Zeiher AM, Drexler H, Saurbier B, et al. Endothelium-mediated coronary blood flow modulation in humans. Effects of age, atherosclerosis, hypercholesterolemia, and hypertension. *J. Clin. Invest.* 1993; 92: 652–62.

[11] Taddei S, Salvetti A. Endothelial dysfunction in essential hypertension: clinical implications. *J. Hypertens.* 2002; 20: 1671–4.

[12] Panza JA, Casino PR, Badar DM, et al. Effect of increased availability of endothelium derived nitric oxide precursor on endothelium-dependent vascular relaxation in normal subjects and in patients with essential hypertension. *Circulation* 1993; 87:1475–81.

[13] Landmesser U, Drexler H. Endothelial function and hypertension. *Curr. Opin. Cardiol.* 2007;22: 316–20.

[14] Higashi Y, Sasaki S, Nakagawa K, Matsuura H, Oshima T, Chayama K. Endothelial function and oxidative stress in renovascular hypertension. *N Engl. J. Med.* 2002; 346: 1954–62.

[15] Redon J, Oliva MR, Tormos C, Giner V, Chaves J, Iradi A, Saez GT. Antioxidant activities and oxidative stress byproducts in human hypertension. *Hypertension* 2003; 41:1096–101.

[16] Touyz RM. Reactive oxygen species, vascular oxidative stress, and redox signaling in hypertension: what is the clinical significance? *Hypertension* 2004; 44: 248–52.

[17] Griendling KK, Sorescu D, Ushio-Fukai M. NAD(P)H oxydase: role in cardiovascular biology and disease. *Circ Res* 2000; 86: 494–501.
[18] Hsueh WA, Wyne K. Renin-Angiotensin-aldosterone system in diabetes and hypertension. *J. Clin. Hypertens.* 2011; 13: 224–37.
[19] Kim S, Iwao H. Molecular and cellular mechanisms of angiotensin II-mediated.
[20] cardiovascular and renal diseases. *Pharmacol. Rev.* 2000: 52: 11–34.
[21] Williams B. Angiotensin II and the pathophysiology of cardiovascular remodeling. *Am. J. Cardiol.* 2001; 87 Suppl 1: S10–17.
[22] Brasier RA, Recinos A, Eledrisi MS. Vascular inflammation and the rennin-angiotensin system. *Arterioscler. Thromb. Vasc. Biol.* 2002; 22: 1257–66.
[23] Duprez DA. Role of the renin-angiotensin-aldosterone system in vascular remodeling and inflammation: a clinical review. *J. Hypertens.* 2006; 24: 983–91.
[24] Watanabe T, Barker TA, Berk BC. Angiotensin II and the endothelium: diverse signals and effects. *Hypertension* 2005; 45: 163–9.
[25] Iwatsubo H, Nagano M et al .Converting enzyme inhibitor improves forearm reactive hyperemia in essential hypertension. *Hypertension*. 1997 Jan;29(1 Pt 2):286-90.
[26] Kabat A, Dhein S. L-arginine supplementation prevents the development of endothelial dysfunction in hyperglycemia. *Pharmacology* 2006; 76: 185–91.
[27] Badimon JJ, Fuster V, Chesebro JH, Badimon L. Coronary atherosclerosis. A multifactorial disease. *Circulation* 1993 Mar;87(3 Suppl):II3-16.
[28] Bondjers G, Glukhova M, Hansson GK, Postnov YV, Reidy MA, Schwartz SM. Hypertension and atherosclerosis. Cause and effect, or two effects with one unknown cause? *Circulation* 1991 Dec;84(6 Suppl):VI2-16.
[29] Fuster V, Badimon JJ, Badimon L. Clinical-pathological correlations of coronary disease progression and regression. *Circulation* 1992 Dec;86(6 Suppl):III1-11.
[30] Landmesser U, Drexler H. The clinical significance of endothelial dysfunction. *Curr. Opin. Cardiol.* 2005 Nov;20(6):547-51.
[31] Vane JR, Anggård EE, Botting RM. Regulatory functions of the vascular endothelium. *N Engl. J. Med.* 1990 Jul 5;323(1):27-36.
[32] Zizek B, Poredos P, Videcnik V. Endothelial dysfunction in hypertensive patients and in normotensive offspring of subjects with essential hypertension. *Heart.* 2001 Feb;85(2):215-7.
[33] Calabrò P, Golia E, Maddaloni V, et al. Adipose tissue-mediated inflammation: the missing link between obesity and cardiovascular disease? Intern Emerg Med.2009 Feb;4(1):25-34. Epub 2008 Dec. Review.
[34] Calabrò P, Limongelli G, Pacileo, et al The role of adiposity as a determinat of an inflammatory milieu. J Cardiovasc Med(Hagerstown). 2008 May;9(5):450-60. Review.
[35] Calabrò P, Limongelli G, Riegler L, et al.Novel insights into the role of cardiotrophin-1 in cardiovascular diseases. *J. Mol. Cell Cardiol*.2009 Feb;46(2):142:8.
[36] De Fronzo RA, Ferrannini E. Insulin resistance. A multifaceted syndrome responsible for NIDDM, obesity, hypertension, dyslipidemia, and atherosclerotic cardiovascular disease. *Diabetes Care.* 1991 Mar;14(3):173-94.
[37] Calabrò P, Chang DW, Willerson Jt, et al. No Release of C-reactive protein in response to inflammatory cytokines by human adipocytes:linking obesity to vascular inflammation. *J. Am. Coll. Cardiolo*. 2005 Sep 20;46(and):1112-3.

[38] Tamakoshi K, Yatsuya H, Kondo T, Hori Y, Ishikawa M, Zhang H, Murata C, Otsuka R, Zhu S, Toyoshima H. The metabolic syndrome is associated with elevated circulating C-reactive protein in healthy reference range, a systemic low-grade inflammatory state. *Int. J. Obes. Relat. Metab. Disord.* 2003 Apr;27(4):443-9.

[39] Olijhoek JK, van der Graaf Y, Banga JD, Algra A, Rabelink TJ, Visseren FL; SMART Study Group. The metabolic syndrome is associated with advanced vascular damage in patients with coronary heart disease, stroke, peripheral arterial disease or abdominal aortic aneurysm. *Eur. Heart J.* 2004 Feb;25(4):342-8.

[40] Pignoli P, Longo T. Ultrasound evaluation of atherosclerosis. Methodological problems and technological developments. *Eur. Surg. Res.* 1986;18(3-4):238-53.

[41] Poredos P. Intima-media thickness: indicator of cardiovascular risk and measure of the extent of atherosclerosis. *Vasc. Med.* 2004 Feb;9(1):46-54.

[42] Poredos P, Orehek M, Tratnik E. Smoking is associated with dose-related increase of intima-media thickness and endothelial dysfunction. *Angiology* 1999 Mar;50(3):201-8.

[43] Salonen JT, Korpela H, Salonen R, Nyyssönen K. Precision and reproducibility of ultrasonographic measurement of progression of common carotid artery atherosclerosis. *Lancet* 1993 May1;341(8853):1158-9.

[44] Zizek B, Poredos P. Dependence of morphological changes of the carotid arteries on essential hypertension and accompanying risk factors. *Int. Angiol.* 2002 Mar;21(1): 70-7.

[45] Tang R, Hennig M, Thomasson B, Scherz R, Ravinetto R, Catalini R, Rubba P, Zanchetti A, Bond MG. Baseline reproducibility of B-mode ultrasonic measurement of carotid artery intima-media thickness: the European Lacidipine Study on Atherosclerosis (ELSA).*J. Hypertens.* 2000 Feb;18(2):197-201.

[46] Glasser SP, Arnett DK, McVeigh GE, Finkelstein SM, Bank AJ, Morgan DJ, Cohn JN. Vascular compliance and cardiovascular disease: a risk factor or a marker? *Am. J. Hypertens* 1997 Oct;10(10 Pt 1):1175-89.

[47] Nichols WW. Clinical measurement of arterial stiffness obtained from noninvasive pressure waveforms. *Am. J. Hypertens.* 2005 Jan;18(1 Pt 2):3S-10S.

[48] Fournier A, El Esper N, Makdassi R, et al. Hypertension and progression of renal insufficiency. *Nephrol. Dial. Transplant.* 1994; 9 Suppl 3: S28–34.

[49] Freedman BI, Iskandar SS, Appel RG. The link between hypertension and nephrosclerosis. *Am. J. Kidney Dis.* 1995; 25: 207–21.

[50] Hill GS. Hypertensive nephrosclerosis. *Curr. Opin. Nephrol. Hypertens.* 2008; 17: 266–70.

[51] Volpe M, Savoia C, De Paolis P, et al. The renin-angiotensin system as a risk factor and therapeutic target for cardiovascular and renal disease. *J. Am. Soc. Nephrol.* 2002; 13 Suppl 3: S173–8.

[52] Momback AS, Toto R. Dual blockade of the renin-angiotensin-aldosterone system: beyond the ACE inhibitor and angiotensin-II receptor blocker combination. *Am. J. Hypertens.* 2009; 22: 1032-40.

[53] Riccioni G. Aliskiren in the treatment of hypertension and organ damage. *Cardiovasc. Ther.* 2011; 29: 77–87.

[54] Ruilope LM, Bakris GL. Renal function and target organ damage in hypertension. *Eur. Heart J. 2011*; 32: 1599–604.

[55] Segura J, Campo C, Gil P, et al. Development of chronic kidney disease and cardiovascular prognosis in essential hypertensive patients. *J. Am. Soc. Nephrol.* 2004; 15: 1616–22.

[56] Meguid El Nahas, A. and Bello, A.K. Chronic kidney disease: the global challenge. *Lancet* 365, 331-340 (2005).

[57] Perr, H.M. et al. Early predictors of 15-year and-stage renal disease in hypertensive patients. *Hypertension* 25, 587-59.

[58] Klag, M.J. et al. Blood pressure and end-stage renal disease in men. *N. Engl. J. Med.* 334, 13-18(1996).

[59] Hill GS. Hypertensive nephrosclerosis. *Curr. Opin. Nephrol. Hypertens.* 2008; 17: 266–70.

[60] Levey AS, Cattran D, Friedman A et al. Proteinuria as a surrogate outcome in CKD: report of a scientific workshop sponsored by national Kidney Foundation and the US Food and Drug Administration. *Am. J. Kidney Dis.* 2009; 54: 205–26.

[61] Ruilope LM, Bakris GL. Renal function and target organ damage in hypertension. *Eur. Heart J. 2011*; 32: 1599–604.

[62] Ibsen H, Olsen MH, Wachtell K et al. Reduction in albuminuria translates to reduction in cardiovascular events in hypertensive patients: Losartan intervention for endpoint reduction in hypertension study. *Hypertension* 2005; 45: 198–202.

[63] Renal outcomes with telmisartan, ramipril, or both, in people at high vascular risk (the ONTARGET study: a multicentre, randomized, double-blind, controlled trial. *The Lancet,* Volume 372, Issue 9638, Pages 547-553, 16 August 2008.

[64] Sanderson JE. Heart failure with a normal ejection fraction. *Heart* 2007; 93: 155–8.

[65] Zile MR, Brutsaert DL. New concepts in diastolic dysfunction and diastolic heart failure: Part I and II: diagnosis, prognosis, and measurements of diastolic function. *Circulation*. 2002; 105: 1387–93, 1503–8.

[66] Bhm M, Reil JC, Bramlage P, Pitt B, Zannad F. Clinical efficacy of aldosterone-blocking agents. *Eur. Heart J.* 2011; 13 Suppl B: B36–9.

[67] Hart CY, Meyer DM, Tazelaar HD, et al. Load versus humoral activation in the genesis of early hypertensive heart disease. *Circulation* 2001; 104: 215–20.

[68] Wang J, Nagueh SF. Current perspectives on cardiac function in patients with diastolic heart failure. *Circulation* 2009; 119: 1146–57.

[69] ML, Salvetti M, Rizzoni D, Monteduro C, Castellano M, Agabiti-Rosei E. Persistence of left ventricular hypertrophy is a stronger indicator of cardiovascular events than baseline left ventricular mass or systolic performance: 10 years of follow-up. *Muiesan. J. Hypertens. Suppl.* 1996 Dec;14(5):S43-9.

[70] Zizek B, Poredos P, Trojar A, Zeljko T. Diastolic dysfunction is associated with insulin resistance, but not with aldosterone level in normotensive offspring of hypertensive families. Cardiology. 2008;111(1):8-15. Epub 2008 Feb 1.

[71] Frohlic ED, Susic D., Pressure overload. *Heart Fail Clin.*2012 Jan;8(1):21-32.

[72] Akki A, Smith K, Seymour AM. Compensated cardiac hypertrophy is characterised by a decline in palmitate oxidation. *Mol. Cell Biochem.* 2008 Apr;311(1-2):215-24.

[73] Akki A, Seymour AM. Western diet impairs metabolic remodelling and contractile efficiency in cardiac hypertrophy. Cardiovasc. Res. 2009 Feb 15;81(3):610-7.

[74] Barry SP, Davidson SM, Townsend PA. Molecular regulation of cardiac hypertrophy. *Int. J. Biochem. Cell Biol.* 2008;40(10):2023-39.

[75] Deschepper CF, Boutin-Ganache I, Zahabi A, Jiang Z. In search of cardiovascular candidate genes: interactions between phenotypes and genotypes. *Hypertension.* 2002 Feb;39(2 Pt 2):332-6.

[76] Brush JE Jr, Cannon RO 3rd, Schenke WH, Bonow RO, Leon MB, Maron BJ, Epstein SE. Angina due to coronary microvascular disease in hypertensive patients without left ventricular hypertrophy. *N Engl. J. Med.*1988 Nov 17;319(20):1302-7.

[77] Kuznetsova T, Staessen JA, Stolarz K, Ryabikov A, Tikhonoff V, Olszanecka A, Bianchi G, Brand E, Casiglia E, Dominiczak A, Fagard R, Malyutina S, Nikitin Y, Kawecka-Jaszcz K. Relationship between left ventricular mass and the ACE D/I polymorphism varies according to sodium intake. European Project On Genes in Hypertension (EPOGH) Investigators. *J. Hypertens.* 2004 Feb;22(2):287-95.

[78] Kozàkovà M, Palombo C, Pratali l, Pittella G, Galetta F, L'Abbate A. Mechanism of coronary flow reserve impairment in human hypertension echocardiography. *Hypertension.* 1997 Feb;29(2):551-9.

[79] Antony I, Nitenberg A, Foult JM, Aptecar E. Coronary vasodilator reserve in untreated and treated hypertensive patients with and without left ventricular hypertrophy. *J. Am. Coll Cardiol.* 1993 Aug;22(2):514-20.

[80] Agabiti-Rosei E, Muiesan ML. Hypertensive left ventricular hypertrophy: pathophysiological and clinical issues. *Blood Press.* 2001;10(5-6):288-98.

[81] Kozàkovà M, Palombo C, Pratali L, Pittella G, Galetta F, L'Abbate A. Mechanisms of coronary flow reserve impairment in human hypertension. An integrated approach by transthoracic and transesophageal echocardiography. *Hypertension.* 1997 Feb;29(2):551-9.

[82] Dahlöf B, Herlitz H, Aurell M, Hansson L. Reversal of cardiovascular structural changes when treating essential hypertension. The importance of the renin-angiotensin-aldosterone system. *Am. J. Hypertens.* 1992 Dec;5(12 Pt 1):900-11.

[83] Oren S, Grossman E, Frohlich ED. Reduction in left ventricular mass in patients with systemic hypertension treated with enalapril, lisinopril, or fosenopril. *Am. J. Cardiol.* 1996 Jan 1;77(1):93-6.

Reviewed by Prof. Davide Cattano, MD. University of Texas, Houston, USA

Index

B

C

D

E

I

J

K

L

M

N

O

P

Q

R

S

T

U

V

W

Y

Z